Wall Pilate For Seniors and Beginners

Strengthen Your Muscles, Stretching Exercises And Improve Your Flexibility With A 28 Day Challenge

Deborah M. Lawis

Contents

Nutritional Tips for Optimal Performance In Wall Pilate

Micronutrient and Their Sources

CONCLUSION

1

INTRODUCTION

What is wall Pilate

Before delving into the specifics of Wall Pilates, it's essential to grasp the fundamentals of Pilates itself. Developed by Joseph Pilates, this exercise regimen initially emerged as a means to aid dancers in recuperating from the repetitive strain injuries inherent in their profession.

Understanding Pilates

Pilates, in its original form, entails a series of exercises performed either on a mat or with the aid of specialized equipment like the reformer. These exercises are meticulously designed to target various muscle groups, fostering muscle toning, strength enhancement, and the expansion of one's range of motion.

Exploring Wall Pilates

Wall Pilates, as an offshoot of traditional Pilates, adopts many of the same foundational movements utilized in mat-based or reformer Pilates routines. However, what distinguishes Wall Pilates is the incorporation of a wall as a supportive element. While exercises such as glute bridges and abdominal crunches remain integral components of the regimen, practitioners replace conventional assisting tools with the wall's surface.

The essence of Wall Pilates lies in its innovative utilization of vertical support, lending a unique dimension to familiar exercises. By harnessing the wall's stability and structure, individuals engage in movements that not only challenge their muscles but also promote proper alignment and form.

In Wall Pilates, the wall serves as both a stabilizing force and a source of resistance, intensifying the efficacy of each exercise. Through subtle modifications and strategic positioning, practitioners leverage the wall's presence to deepen stretches, refine movements, and enhance overall performance.

Moreover, Wall Pilates fosters versatility by offering a dynamic range of exercises adaptable to varying fitness levels and objectives. Whether aiming to bolster core strength, improve flexibility, or enhance overall well-being, individuals can tailor their Wall Pilates practice to suit their specific goals and preferences.

While rooted in the principles of traditional Pilates, Wall Pilates introduces a novel approach by integrating the vertical support of a wall. This fusion of stability, resistance, and versatility defines the essence of Wall Pilates, offering practitioners a refreshing perspective on this time-honored exercise discipline.

Why is it different from classic Pilate

The divergence between Wall Pilates and classic Pilates stems from the innovative incorporation of the wall as a fundamental component of the exercise regimen. While both disciplines share a common foundation rooted in Joseph Pilates' principles, Wall Pilates introduces a distinctive dimension through the utilization of vertical support. Let's delve deeper into the key distinctions that set Wall Pilates apart from its traditional counterpart:

Inclusion of Vertical Support:

- Classic Pilates predominantly relies on exercises performed on a mat or specialized equipment like the reformer, focusing on developing core strength, flexibility, and overall body awareness.
- In contrast, Wall Pilates integrates the vertical surface of a wall into its repertoire, offering practitioners a stable support system to enhance alignment, stability, and engagement of muscles. This vertical support serves as a guiding force, aiding individuals in maintaining proper form and posture throughout each movement.

Variation in Assisting Tools:

- Classic Pilates exercises often utilize mats, resistance springs, and other equipment to facilitate movements and provide resistance.
- In Wall Pilates, the wall itself serves as the primary assisting tool, replacing conventional equipment with its stable surface. This substitution not only offers a unique tactile experience but also encourages practitioners to adapt familiar exercises to leverage the wall's support and resistance.

Emphasis on Alignment and Stability:

- While both disciplines prioritize proper alignment and stability, Wall Pilates places particular emphasis on utilizing the wall to refine these aspects.
- The vertical orientation of the wall serves as a visual and tactile reference point, guiding individuals to maintain correct posture and alignment throughout each exercise. By leveraging the wall's support, practitioners can deepen their awareness of body mechanics, fostering a greater sense of stability and control.

Enhanced Intensity and Challenge:

- Wall Pilates introduces an added dimension of intensity and challenge through the incorporation of the wall's resistance.
- By leveraging the wall's stability and structure, practitioners can intensify exercises, effectively engaging targeted muscle groups and enhancing overall strength and endurance. This heightened level of challenge offers practitioners an opportunity to push their boundaries and progress in their fitness journey.

Accessibility and Adaptability:

- While classic Pilates may require specialized equipment and training, Wall Pilates offers a more accessible and adaptable approach to exercise.
- With minimal equipment requirements and the flexibility to practice in various settings, Wall Pilates provides individuals with the opportunity to incorporate Pilates principles into their daily routines. Additionally, the versatility of Wall Pilates exercises allows for modifications to accommodate different fitness levels and goals, making it suitable for a wide range of practitioners.

The integration of the wall as a supportive element distinguishes Wall Pilates from classic Pilates, offering practitioners a fresh perspective on this time-honored exercise discipline. By harnessing the benefits of vertical support, Wall Pilates empowers individuals to enhance their alignment, stability, and strength while exploring new dimensions of movement and mindfulness.

What are the advantages of wall Pilates

Many individuals are initially drawn to Pilates due to its potential to address various health concerns, such as Osteoporosis or arthritis, prompting them to embark on this exercise journey. Renowned for its ability to enhance bone density, Pilates is revered for its bone-strengthening properties. Wall Pilates, characterized by its gentle nature and minimal risk of injury, presents a compelling option for individuals seeking to fortify their skeletal health. Through consistent practice, Wall Pilates offers the promise of bolstering bone mass, thereby mitigating the risk of bone-related ailments.

Wall Pilates serves as an effective means of elongating the spine and promoting optimal spinal alignment, setting it apart as an invaluable tool for enhancing postural integrity. By placing emphasis on targeting the abdominal, gluteal, and back muscles, Wall Pilates facilitates the strengthening of core muscles while mitigating unfavorable spinal curvature. As practitioners achieve greater spinal alignment and core strength, they experience relief from backaches and stiffness, paving the way for improved posture and enhanced overall well-being.

Expectant mothers stand to reap significant benefits from incorporating Wall Pilates into their fitness routine, particularly as they navigate the different stages of pregnancy. Not only does Wall Pilates offer a means of adapting to the physical changes associated with pregnancy, but it also aids in preparing the body for childbirth. Often complemented by breathing exercises, Wall Pilates provides expectant mothers with a sanctuary for stress relief and relaxation. Furthermore, the adaptability of Pilates exercises ensures that intensity levels can be tailored to meet the unique needs of each individual throughout pregnancy.

Wall Pilates holds promise in alleviating menstrual cramps by targeting the lower back muscles and pelvis, thereby offering relief from discomfort. By elongating and opening these areas, Wall Pilates contributes to improved circulation and reduced inflammation in the pelvic floor region. Strengthening the pelvic floor muscles not only enhances bladder control but also fosters increased sexual satisfaction, thus promoting overall well-being.

Beyond its physical benefits, Wall Pilates offers profound psychological advantages, including enhanced sleep quality. Through a combination of stress-relieving techniques inherent in Wall Pilates and deep breathing exercises, individuals experience improvements in both the quantity and quality of their sleep. This holistic approach to well-being addresses both physical and mental aspects, fostering a sense of balance and tranquility.

One of the standout benefits of Wall Pilates lies in its provision of instantaneous feedback, offering practitioners a unique perspective compared to traditional mat-based Pilates. The wall serves as a reliable support system for the back, hips, and shoulders, facilitating proper alignment and stability throughout each movement. This feedback mechanism not only enhances the efficacy of exercises but also promotes a deeper understanding of body mechanics, further enhancing the overall Pilates experience.

Benefits Highlights:

- Enhanced bone density and skeletal health
- Improved spinal alignment and posture
- Strengthening of core muscles and reduction of backaches
- Adaptability for pregnant individuals, aiding in preparation for childbirth

- Alleviation of menstrual cramps and promotion of pelvic floor health
- Enhanced sleep quality and stress relief

- Instantaneous feedback and deeper understanding of body mechanics

2

WHAT YOU REALLY NEED

Equipment and tools

For Beginners and Seniors:

Sturdy Wall: The primary requirement for Wall Pilates is a stable and clean wall space, preferably free from obstructions, to serve as a supportive surface for various exercises.

Yoga Mat or Comfortable Flooring: While not essential, a yoga mat or padded flooring can enhance comfort and stability during floor-based exercises, providing cushioning for joints and spine.

Comfortable Clothing: Wear breathable and stretchy clothing that allows for unrestricted movement during the practice, ensuring comfort and ease of movement.

Optional Props for Added Challenge: Consider incorporating props such as resistance bands, hand weights, or Pilates balls for added variety and challenge to your routine, providing options for progressive difficulty.

Water Bottle and Towel: Stay hydrated and comfortable during your workout by keeping a water bottle and towel nearby to wipe away sweat and maintain hydration.

Additional Equipment Adaptations for Seniors:

Chair or Stability Ball for Support: Seniors may benefit from using a sturdy chair or stability ball for added support and balance during exercises, particularly for standing or seated movements.

Gentle Resistance Bands: Choose gentle resistance bands with varying levels of resistance to accommodate different fitness levels and abilities, providing gentle strengthening for muscles and joints.

Padded Mat or Cushioning: Use a padded exercise mat or additional cushioning to provide support and comfort during floor-based exercises, reducing pressure on sensitive joints.

Gradual Progression and Modifications: Start with basic exercises and gradually progress to more challenging movements, providing modifications as needed to accommodate physical limitations or mobility issues.

Personalized Guidance and Supervision: Seek personalized guidance from a qualified Pilates instructor or physical therapist, especially for seniors with specific health concerns, to ensure exercises are performed safely and effectively.

By adhering to these equipment recommendations and adaptations, beginners and seniors can enjoy a safe and effective Wall Pilates practice tailored to their individual needs and abilities, promoting strength, flexibility, and overall well-being.

Space requirement and practice area

For those unable to invest in a dedicated wall unit, an accessible alternative is the popular Wall Pilates routine, requiring nothing more than the four walls of your home. This version of Wall Pilates offers a practical solution, utilizing minimal equipment to maximize your workout experience.

Here's a breakdown of the essential Wall Pilates equipment to optimize your routine:

- **Yoga Mat:** A fundamental component, the yoga mat provides essential cushioning for your back against hard flooring, ensuring comfort during floor-based exercises.

- **Resistance Bands:** These versatile tools are invaluable for building muscle and enhancing resistance in various workouts, including Pilates. They add a dynamic element to exercises, intensifying muscle engagement and challenging your strength.

- **Pilates Ball:** Offering versatility and increased challenge, the Pilates ball is a valuable addition to your equipment arsenal. It amplifies the difficulty of traditional exercises and can be utilized for core-targeting workouts, lower body exercises, wall planks, push-ups, as well as extension and stretching movements.

- **Ankle Weights:** Enhancing lower body strength, ankle weights provide additional resistance to leg-focused exercises, aiding in muscle development and toning.

What Is the Best Wall Pilates Equipment?

In studio settings, the most essential Wall Pilates equipment includes dedicated wall units and well-padded yoga mats. Wall units offer versatility for a wide range of exercises, while quality yoga mats ensure comfort and support during floor routines.

For individuals opting to practice Wall Pilates at home without access to a wall unit, a high-quality yoga mat suffices, along with any available wall space. While weights, resistance bands, and Pilates balls serve as beneficial enhancements, they are not essential for a fulfilling Wall Pilates experience.

Set Your Goals

Setting goals and achieving them is a multifaceted process that requires careful planning, dedication, and perseverance. Here's a comprehensive guide to help you set and attain your goals effectively:

Define Your Goals:

Start by clearly defining your goals. Make them specific, measurable, achievable, relevant, and time-bound (SMART). For example, instead of saying, "I want to improve my fitness," specify, "I aim to practice Wall Pilates three times a week for the next three months to enhance my core strength and flexibility."

Break Down Your Goals:

Break down your overarching goal into smaller, manageable tasks or milestones. This makes the goal less daunting and allows you to track your progress more effectively. Create a timeline with deadlines for each milestone to stay accountable.

Identify Potential Obstacles:

Anticipate potential obstacles or challenges that may hinder your progress. This could include time constraints, lack of motivation, or unforeseen circumstances. By identifying these barriers in advance, you can develop strategies to overcome them proactively.

Develop a Plan of Action:

Create a detailed plan of action outlining the specific steps you need to take to achieve your goals. This may include scheduling your Wall Pilates sessions, setting aside dedicated time for practice, and identifying resources or support systems to help you along the way.

Stay Motivated:

Find sources of motivation to keep you inspired and focused on your goals. This could involve setting rewards for achieving milestones, finding a workout buddy to keep you accountable, or visualizing the benefits of achieving your goals.

Track Your Progress:

Monitor your progress regularly to stay on track and identify areas for improvement. Keep a journal or use tracking tools to record your workouts, measure your performance, and celebrate your achievements along the way.

Adjust and Adapt:

Be flexible and willing to adjust your approach as needed. If you encounter setbacks or obstacles, reassess your goals and modify your plan accordingly. Remember that setbacks are a natural part of the process, and learning from them will ultimately make you stronger and more resilient.

Stay Consistent:

Consistency is key to achieving any goal. Make a commitment to yourself to stay consistent with your Wall Pilates practice, even on days when you don't feel motivated. Remember that small, consistent efforts over time lead to significant results.

Seek Support and Accountability:

Surround yourself with a supportive community of friends, family, or fellow practitioners who can cheer you on and hold you accountable. Share your goals with others and enlist their support to help you stay motivated and committed to your journey.

Celebrate Your Achievements:

Finally, celebrate your achievements and milestones along the way. Acknowledge your progress and the hard work you've put in to reach your goals. Celebrating your successes will not only boost your morale but also reinforce your commitment to continued growth and success.

By following these steps and remaining dedicated to your goals, you can set yourself up for success and achieve your desired outcomes in Wall Pilates or any other endeavor you pursue. Remember that goal setting is a dynamic process, and staying adaptable and resilient in the face of challenges will ultimately lead to long-term success.

3

SAFETY AND PRECAUTIONS

nsuring safety during Wall Pilates practice is paramount, especially for beginners and seniors who may be more susceptible to injuries or physical limitations. Here's an extensive guide covering 10 safety precautions for Wall Pilates tailored to both beginners and seniors:

Safety Precautions for Seniors:

Consult with a Healthcare Professional: Before starting any new exercise program, seniors should consult with their healthcare provider to ensure that Wall Pilates is safe for their individual health condition. A thorough assessment can help identify any potential risks or contraindications and provide guidance on appropriate exercise modifications.

Start Slowly and Progress Gradually: Seniors should begin their Wall Pilates practice at a comfortable pace and gradually increase the intensity and duration of their workouts over time. This gradual progression allows the body to adapt to the demands of exercise and reduces the risk of overexertion or injury.

Focus on Proper Alignment and Form: Proper alignment and form are crucial for preventing injuries in seniors. Focus on maintaining a neutral spine, engaging the core muscles, and moving with control and precision during each exercise. Avoid overextending or straining the body, especially in vulnerable areas such as the spine and joints.

Use Supportive Props and Equipment: Seniors may benefit from using supportive props such as yoga blocks, straps, or pillows to assist with balance, stability, and alignment during Wall Pilates exercises. These props can help reduce strain on the body and provide added support where needed.

Listen to Your Body: Seniors should listen to their bodies and pay attention to any signs of discomfort, pain, or fatigue during exercise. If something doesn't feel right, it's important to stop and rest or modify the exercise as needed. Pushing through pain can lead to injury and should be avoided.

Stay Hydrated and Well-Nourished: Proper hydration and nutrition are essential for seniors engaging in exercise. Drink plenty of water before, during, and after your Wall Pilates session to stay hydrated and support muscle function. Additionally, maintain a balanced diet rich in nutrients to support overall health and vitality.

Avoid Overexertion and Fatigue: Seniors should be mindful of their energy levels and avoid overexerting themselves during Wall Pilates practice. Pace yourself, take breaks as needed, and prioritize rest and recovery to prevent fatigue and burnout. Listen to your body's cues and adjust your workout intensity accordingly.

Choose Low-Impact Exercises: Opt for low-impact exercises that are gentle on the joints and muscles, especially if you have pre-existing health conditions or mobility limitations. Focus on controlled movements that promote joint mobility, stability, and flexibility without causing undue strain or discomfort.

Warm Up and Cool Down Properly: Always include a thorough warm-up and cool-down routine before and after your Wall Pilates session. A proper warm-up prepares the body for exercise by increasing blood flow to the muscles and reducing the risk of injury. Similarly, cooling down helps to gradually lower heart rate, stretch tight muscles, and promote relaxation.

Seek Professional Guidance: Consider working with a certified Pilates instructor or physical therapist who has experience working with seniors. They can provide personalized instruction, guidance, and support to help you safely and effectively incorporate Wall Pilates into your fitness routine.

Safety Precautions for Beginners:

Start with a Beginner-Friendly Program: Beginners should start with a beginner-friendly Wall Pilates program that focuses on foundational movements and basic exercises. Avoid jumping into advanced workouts before mastering the fundamentals to reduce the risk of injury.

Learn Proper Technique: Proper technique is essential for beginners to safely and effectively perform Wall Pilates exercises. Take the time to learn proper alignment, breathing techniques, and movement patterns under the guidance of a qualified instructor or through instructional videos and resources.

Engage Core Muscles: Focus on engaging the core muscles throughout your Wall Pilates practice to provide stability and support for the spine and pelvis. Core engagement helps prevent excessive strain on the lower back and promotes proper alignment during exercises.

Use Props for Support: Beginners may benefit from using props such as yoga blocks, straps, or resistance bands to provide support and assistance during exercises. These props can help improve alignment, enhance stability, and reduce the risk of injury while building strength and flexibility.

Start Slowly and Progress Gradually: Beginners should start their Wall Pilates practice at a slow and manageable pace, gradually increasing the intensity and duration of their workouts as they build strength, flexibility, and confidence. Rushing into advanced exercises can lead to injury and should be avoided.

Listen to Your Body: Pay attention to your body's signals and avoid pushing yourself beyond your limits. If you experience pain, discomfort, or fatigue during exercise, take a break and reassess your approach. Honor your body's needs and modify exercises as needed to prevent injury.

Stay Hydrated and Well-Nourished: Proper hydration and nutrition are essential for supporting your body's energy levels and recovery during Wall Pilates practice. Drink plenty of water before, during, and after your workouts, and fuel your body with nutritious foods to support optimal performance.

Warm Up and Cool Down Properly: Always start your Wall Pilates session with a thorough warm-up to prepare your body for exercise and reduce the risk of injury. Likewise, incorporate a cool-down routine at the end of your workout to stretch tight muscles, lower your heart rate, and promote relaxation.

Avoid Overexertion: Beginners should avoid overexerting themselves during Wall Pilates practice, especially in the early stages of learning. Pace yourself, take breaks as needed, and focus on quality over quantity in your movements. Pushing too hard can lead to burnout and injury.

Seek Instruction and Guidance: Consider taking beginner-level Wall Pilates classes or working with a certified instructor who can provide personalized instruction and guidance. A qualified instructor can help you learn proper technique, choose appropriate exercises, and progress safely in your practice.

4

WARM-UP AND COOLING DOWN

The Importance of warm-up

Warm-up exercises are an essential component of any workout routine, including Wall Pilates, particularly for beginners and seniors. A proper warm-up serves several crucial purposes that contribute to the safety, effectiveness, and overall enjoyment of the Pilates practice.

1. Prepares the Body for Movement:

The primary purpose of a warm-up is to prepare the body for physical activity by gradually increasing blood flow to the muscles, ligaments, and tendons. This increased blood flow delivers oxygen and nutrients to the muscles, enhancing their ability to contract and relax efficiently during exercise.

2. Reduces the Risk of Injury:

Engaging in a comprehensive warm-up routine helps reduce the risk of injury by gradually increasing body temperature and improving joint mobility and flexibility. Warm muscles and joints are more pliable and less prone to strain or tears, making it safer to perform the dynamic movements associated with Wall Pilates.

3. Improves Muscle Elasticity and Flexibility:

Warm-up exercises promote muscle elasticity and flexibility, allowing for greater range of motion and fluidity of movement during Pilates practice. This increased flexibility not only enhances performance but also reduces the likelihood of muscle strains or injuries resulting from overstretching.

4. Enhances Joint Lubrication:

Gentle warm-up movements stimulate the production of synovial fluid in the joints, which serves as a lubricant to reduce friction and facilitate smooth movement. Improved joint lubrication helps maintain joint health and function, especially in seniors who may experience stiffness or reduced mobility.

5. Activates Neuromuscular Pathways:

Warm-up exercises activate neuromuscular pathways between the brain and muscles, enhancing coordination, balance, and proprioception. This neural activation primes the body for more precise and controlled movements during Wall Pilates, reducing the risk of falls or accidents, particularly in seniors.

6. Enhances Mental Preparedness:

A warm-up routine provides an opportunity to mentally prepare for the upcoming Pilates practice, helping to focus the mind and cultivate mindfulness. Taking a few moments to connect with the breath, center the mind, and set intentions for the session can enhance concentration and promote a deeper mind-body connection.

7. Gradually Increases Intensity:

Gradually increasing the intensity of warm-up exercises allows the body to transition from a state of rest to one of physical exertion gradually. This progressive approach prevents shock to the cardiovascular system and prepares the body for the higher intensity movements and challenges of Wall Pilates.

8. Promotes Relaxation and Stress Reduction:

Warm-up exercises provide an opportunity to release tension and stress accumulated throughout the day, promoting relaxation and mental clarity. Incorporating gentle stretching, deep breathing, and mindfulness techniques into the warm-up routine can help calm the nervous system and reduce anxiety or tension.

9. Facilitates Mind-Body Connection:

Warm-up exercises serve as a bridge between the mind and body, facilitating a deeper connection and awareness of physical sensations, movement patterns, and alignment. This heightened mind-body connection is essential for performing Pilates exercises with precision, control, and mindfulness.

10. Sets the Tone for the Workout:

Finally, a well-executed warm-up sets the tone for the entire Wall Pilates workout, establishing a positive and focused mindset and laying the foundation for a successful and enjoyable practice session. By investing time and attention into the warm-up, beginners and seniors can maximize the benefits of their Pilates practice and optimize their overall well-being.

The importance of warm-up in Wall Pilates for both beginners and seniors cannot be overstated. From injury prevention and improved flexibility to enhanced mental preparedness and mind-body connection, a thorough warm-up routine sets the stage for a safe, effective, and rewarding Pilates experience. Incorporating targeted warm-up exercises tailored to the specific needs and abilities of beginners and seniors is essential for maximizing the benefits and enjoyment of Wall Pilates practice.

WARM-UP EXERCISE

Wall Hamstrings Stretch

Starting Position:

- Begin by lying on your back on the floor with your buttocks close to a wall.
- Extend your legs upward, resting them against the wall so that your heels are pointing towards the ceiling.
- Your body should form an L-shape, with your hips and knees at approximately 90-degree angles.

Movement:

- Slowly begin to straighten your legs, pressing your heels towards the ceiling.
- Engage your core muscles to maintain stability and support your lower back.

Positioning:

- Keep your legs straight and toes pointing towards the ceiling throughout the stretch.
- Avoid locking your knees, maintaining a slight bend to prevent strain on the joints.
- Relax your shoulders and neck, allowing them to sink into the floor.

Execution:

- Gently push through your heels to increase the stretch in your hamstrings.
- You should feel a gentle pulling sensation along the back of your legs.
- Hold the stretch for 30 seconds to 2 minutes, breathing deeply and evenly throughout.
- If you experience any discomfort or pain, ease off the stretch immediately and return to a comfortable position.

Time:

- Aim to hold the Wall Hamstrings Stretch for at least 30 seconds to allow the muscles to lengthen and relax.
- For a deeper stretch, you can gradually increase the hold time up to 2 minutes, focusing on maintaining proper form and breathing rhythm.

Tips:

- Avoid overstretching or forcing your legs into a position that feels uncomfortable.
- If you have tight hamstrings or limited flexibility, you may need to bend your knees slightly or adjust the distance between your body and the wall.
- Focus on relaxing into the stretch and releasing any tension or resistance in the muscles.

- Incorporate the Wall Hamstrings Stretch into your warm-up or cooldown routine to improve flexibility and reduce the risk of injury during other activities.
- Listen to your body and modify the stretch as needed to accommodate your individual flexibility and comfort level.

Wall Cat-Cow

Starting Position:

- Begin by standing with your back against a wall, feet hip-width apart, and arms relaxed by your sides.
- Ensure that your head, shoulders, and buttocks are in contact with the wall, maintaining a neutral spine.

Movement:

- Inhale deeply as you slowly slide your hands up the wall, reaching overhead while keeping your arms straight.
- Exhale as you reverse the movement, sliding your hands back down the wall towards your sides.

Positioning:

- Throughout the movement, focus on maintaining contact between your head, shoulders, lower back, and buttocks against the wall.
- Keep your core engaged to stabilize your spine and pelvis.

Execution:

- Move slowly and mindfully, coordinating your breath with the movement of your arms.
- Visualize elongating your spine as you reach your hands up the wall, and then gently return to the starting position as you exhale.
- Repeat the movement for several repetitions, aiming for smooth, controlled motion.

Time:

- Perform the Wall Cat-Cow exercise for 8-10 repetitions, or as many as feels comfortable.
- Focus on the quality of movement and maintaining proper alignment throughout each repetition.

Benefits:

- The Wall Cat-Cow exercise helps to mobilize the spine, improve spinal flexibility, and relieve tension in the back and shoulders.
- By coordinating breath with movement, it encourages relaxation and mindfulness, promoting a sense of calm and well-being.
- This exercise can also help to improve posture and alleviate stiffness or discomfort associated

with prolonged sitting or standing.

Tips:

- Focus on moving with awareness and intention, paying attention to how each part of your body feels as you perform the exercise.
- If you experience any discomfort or strain, reduce the range of motion or intensity of the movement.
- Incorporate the Wall Cat-Cow exercise into your daily routine as a gentle way to stretch and release tension in the spine and shoulders, particularly if you spend long periods sitting or standing.

Wall Heel Slides

Starting Position:

- Lie on your back on the floor with your buttocks close to a wall.
- Extend your legs upward, resting them against the wall so that your heels are pointing towards the ceiling.
- Your arms should be relaxed by your sides with palms facing down.

Movement:

- Slowly slide one heel down the wall towards the floor, keeping the leg straight but not locked.
- Pause when you feel a gentle stretch in the back of your leg, then return the heel to the starting position.
- Repeat the movement with the opposite leg, alternating sides.

Positioning:

- Maintain contact between your lower back and the floor throughout the movement to stabilize your pelvis.
- Keep your core engaged to support your lower back and prevent excessive arching.

Execution:

- Move slowly and with control, focusing on the sensation of the stretch in the back of your legs.
- Avoid bouncing or jerking movements, as this can strain the muscles and joints.
- As you become more comfortable with the exercise, you can gradually increase the range of motion of the heel slide.

Time:

- Perform 8-10 repetitions of the Wall Heel Slides on each leg, or as many as feels comfortable.
- Aim for smooth, controlled movement and focus on maintaining proper form throughout.

Benefits:

- The Wall Heel Slides exercise helps to stretch the hamstrings and calf muscles, improving flexibility and reducing tension in the lower body.
- It also promotes mobility in the hip and knee joints, which can be beneficial for individuals who spend long periods sitting or standing.
- By strengthening the muscles around the knees and ankles, it may also help to improve stability and reduce the risk of injury during physical activity.

Tips:

- Focus on breathing deeply and evenly throughout the exercise to promote relaxation and enhance the effectiveness of the stretch.
- If you experience any discomfort or pain, reduce the range of motion of the heel slide or stop the exercise altogether.
- Incorporate the Wall Heel Slides into your regular stretching routine to improve flexibility and reduce muscle tension in the lower body.

Wall Arm Circles

Starting Position:

- Stand with your back against a wall, feet hip-width apart, and arms relaxed by your sides.
- Ensure that your head, shoulders, and buttocks are in contact with the wall, maintaining a neutral spine.

Movement:

- Begin by lifting your arms out to the sides until they are parallel to the floor, forming a T-shape with your body.
- Keeping your arms straight, slowly make circular motions with your arms, moving them forward in a circular motion.
- Continue circling your arms forward for several repetitions, then reverse the motion, circling your arms backward.

Positioning:

- Maintain contact between your head, shoulders, and buttocks against the wall throughout the exercise.
- Keep your core engaged to stabilize your spine and pelvis, preventing excessive arching or leaning forward.

Execution:

- Move your arms in a slow, controlled manner, focusing on the quality of the movement rather than speed.
- Visualize drawing large circles with your fingertips, engaging the muscles of the shoulders and upper back.

- Breathe deeply and rhythmically as you perform the arm circles, coordinating your breath with the movement.

Time:

- Perform 8-10 repetitions of the Wall Arm Circles in each direction, or as many as feels comfortable.
- Aim for smooth, fluid motion and focus on maintaining proper alignment and posture throughout.

Benefits:

- Wall Arm Circles help to improve shoulder mobility and flexibility, reducing stiffness and tension in the muscles of the upper back and shoulders.
- By engaging the muscles of the arms and upper back, this exercise also helps to strengthen and tone these muscle groups, promoting better posture and alignment.
- The controlled, circular motion of the arms can help to increase blood flow to the muscles, enhancing circulation and promoting relaxation.

Variations:

- For individuals with limited shoulder mobility or flexibility, you can perform smaller circles with your arms to reduce the intensity of the exercise.

- To add an extra challenge, you can hold a light weight in each hand while performing the arm circles, increasing resistance and muscle engagement.

Tips:

- Focus on maintaining proper alignment and posture throughout the exercise, keeping your spine neutral and your shoulders relaxed.
- If you experience any discomfort or pain during the arm circles, reduce the range of motion or stop the exercise altogether.
- Incorporate the Wall Arm Circles into your warm-up routine to prepare the shoulders and upper back for more strenuous activity, or use them as a gentle stretching exercise to relieve tension and promote relaxation.

Wall Lateral Arm Raises

Starting Position:

- Stand with your back against a wall, feet hip-width apart, and arms relaxed by your sides.
- Ensure that your head, shoulders, and buttocks are in contact with the wall, maintaining a neutral spine.

Movement:

- Begin by lifting both arms out to the sides until they are parallel to the floor, forming a T-shape with your body.

- Keep your arms straight and palms facing downward throughout the movement.
- Slowly lower your arms back down to the starting position with control.

Positioning:

- Maintain contact between your head, shoulders, and buttocks against the wall throughout the exercise.
- Keep your core engaged to stabilize your spine and pelvis, preventing excessive arching or leaning forward.

Execution:

- Move your arms in a slow, controlled manner, focusing on engaging the muscles of the shoulders and upper back.
- Avoid shrugging your shoulders or tensing your neck muscles during the movement.
- Breathe deeply and rhythmically as you perform the lateral arm raises, coordinating your breath with the movement.

Time:

- Perform 8-10 repetitions of the Wall Lateral Arm Raises, or as many as feels comfortable.

Benefits:

- Wall Lateral Arm Raises help to strengthen and tone the muscles of the shoulders, upper back, and arms.
- By engaging these muscle groups, this exercise can improve shoulder stability and reduce the risk of injury during daily activities.
- The controlled movement of the arms also helps to increase blood flow to the muscles, enhancing circulation and promoting relaxation.

Tips:

- Focus on maintaining proper alignment and posture throughout the exercise, keeping your spine neutral and your shoulders relaxed.
- Keep your movements smooth and controlled, avoiding any jerky or sudden motions.
- If you experience any discomfort or pain during the lateral arm raises, reduce the range of motion or stop the exercise altogether.
- Incorporate the Wall Lateral Arm Raises into your upper body strength training routine to target the muscles of the shoulders, upper back, and arms effectively.

Wall Leg Lifts

Starting Position:

- Lie on your back on the floor with your buttocks close to a wall.
- Extend your legs upward, resting them against the wall so that your heels are pointing towards the ceiling.
- Place your arms by your sides, palms facing down for stability.

Movement:

- Engage your core muscles to stabilize your pelvis and lower back.
- Slowly lift one leg off the wall, keeping it straight and parallel to the floor.
- Hold the lifted position briefly, then lower the leg back towards the wall with control.
- Repeat the movement with the opposite leg, alternating sides.

Positioning:

- Maintain contact between your lower back and the floor throughout the exercise to stabilize your pelvis.
- Keep your core engaged to support your spine and prevent excessive arching.
- Ensure that your legs remain straight and aligned with your hips throughout the movement.

Execution:

- Move slowly and with control, focusing on engaging the muscles of the lower abdomen and thighs.
- Avoid lifting the leg higher than parallel to the floor to prevent strain on the lower back.
- Breathe deeply and rhythmically as you perform the leg lifts, exhaling as you lift the leg and inhaling as you lower it.

Time:

- Perform 8-10 repetitions of the Wall Leg Lifts on each leg, or as many as feels comfortable.

Benefits:

- Wall Leg Lifts target the muscles of the lower abdomen, hips, and thighs, helping to strengthen and tone these muscle groups.
- By engaging the core muscles, this exercise can help improve stability and support proper alignment of the spine and pelvis.
- The controlled movement of the legs helps to increase blood flow to the muscles, promoting circulation and reducing stiffness and tension.

Tips:

- Focus on maintaining proper alignment and posture throughout the exercise, keeping your spine neutral and your shoulders relaxed.
- If you experience any discomfort or pain during the leg lifts, reduce the range of motion or stop the exercise altogether.

- Incorporate the Wall Leg Lifts into your regular strength training routine to target the muscles of the lower abdomen, hips, and thighs, and improve overall lower body strength and stability.

Wall Chest Openers

Starting Position:

- Stand upright facing a wall with your feet hip-width apart and arms relaxed by your sides.
- Position yourself about arm's length away from the wall, ensuring that your feet are firmly planted on the ground.

Movement:

- Reach your arms out to the sides and place your palms flat against the wall at shoulder height, fingers pointing upwards.
- Slowly begin to lean your body forward, keeping your arms extended and palms pressed against the wall.
- Continue to lean forward until you feel a gentle stretch across the front of your chest and shoulders.
- Hold the stretched position for a few breaths, then slowly return to the starting position.

Positioning:

- Keep your head, shoulders, and hips aligned throughout the movement, avoiding any excessive arching or rounding of the spine.
- Engage your core muscles to maintain stability and support your lower back.

Execution:

- Move slowly and with control, focusing on the sensation of the stretch in your chest and shoulders.
- Avoid locking your elbows or straining the muscles of the neck and upper back.
- Breathe deeply and rhythmically as you hold the stretch, allowing the tension in your chest and shoulders to gradually release.

Time:

- Hold the Wall Chest Openers stretch for 20-30 seconds, or longer if you feel comfortable.

Benefits:

- Wall Chest Openers help to stretch the muscles of the chest, shoulders, and front of the arms, which can become tight and tense due to poor posture or prolonged sitting.
- By opening up the chest and shoulders, this exercise can improve posture, reduce rounded

shoulders, and alleviate tension in the upper body.

- The gentle stretch provided by Wall Chest Openers can also help relieve discomfort associated with conditions such as tight pectoral muscles or shoulder impingement.

Tips:

- Focus on maintaining a relaxed and steady breathing pattern throughout the stretch, inhaling deeply as you lean into the stretch and exhaling fully as you release.
- If you experience any discomfort or pain during the stretch, ease off slightly or adjust the position of your arms to reduce the intensity.
- Incorporate Wall Chest Openers into your daily routine to counteract the effects of prolonged sitting and promote better posture and shoulder mobility over time.

Wall Piriformis Stretch

Starting Position:

- Lie on your back on the floor with your buttocks close to a wall.
- Extend your legs upward, resting them against the wall so that your heels are pointing towards the ceiling.
- Your body should form an L-shape, with your hips and knees at approximately 90-degree angles.

Movement:

- Cross one ankle over the opposite knee, forming a figure-four shape with your legs.
- Keep the foot of the crossed leg flexed to protect the knee joint.
- Slowly slide the foot of the crossed leg down the wall until you feel a gentle stretch in the outer hip and buttock of that leg.
- Hold the stretch for the desired duration, then return to the starting position and repeat on the opposite side.

Positioning:

- Keep your head, shoulders, and lower back flat against the floor throughout the stretch to stabilize your pelvis.
- Engage your core muscles to support your spine and prevent excessive arching.

Execution:

- Move slowly and with control, focusing on the sensation of the stretch in the outer hip and buttock.
- Avoid bouncing or jerking movements, as this can strain the muscles and joints.
- Breathe deeply and rhythmically as you hold the stretch, allowing

the tension in your hip and buttock to gradually release.

Time:

- Hold the Wall Piriformis Stretch for 20-30 seconds on each side, or longer if you feel comfortable.
- Aim for a total of 2-3 repetitions on each side, gradually increasing the duration of each stretch as your flexibility improves.

Benefits:

- The Wall Piriformis Stretch targets the piriformis muscle, which can become tight and tense due to prolonged sitting, running, or other activities.
- By stretching the piriformis muscle, this exercise can help alleviate discomfort associated with piriformis syndrome, sciatica, or general hip and buttock tightness.
- The gentle stretch provided by the Wall Piriformis Stretch can also help improve hip mobility and reduce the risk of injury during physical activity.

Tips:

- Focus on relaxing into the stretch and allowing the tension in your hip and buttock to gradually release.
- If you experience any discomfort or pain during the stretch, ease off slightly or adjust the position

of your legs to reduce the intensity.
- Incorporate the Wall Piriformis Stretch into your regular stretching routine to improve hip mobility, reduce tension, and alleviate discomfort in the hip and buttock area.

Wall Neck Rolls

Starting Position:

- Stand tall with your back against a wall, feet shoulder-width apart, and arms relaxed by your sides.
- Ensure that your head, shoulders, and buttocks are in contact with the wall, maintaining a neutral spine.

Movement:

- Slowly lower your chin towards your chest, allowing your head to gently roll forward.
- From this position, begin to roll your head to one side, bringing your ear towards your shoulder.
- Continue the circular motion, rolling your head back, and then towards the opposite shoulder.
- Complete the circle by bringing your chin back to your chest.
- Reverse the direction of the roll, starting by bringing your chin back to your chest and then rolling your head to the opposite side.

Positioning:

- Maintain contact between your head, shoulders, and buttocks against the wall throughout the exercise.
- Keep your shoulders relaxed and avoid shrugging them towards your ears.

Execution:

- Move slowly and with control, focusing on the sensation of the stretch in your neck and shoulders.
- Avoid forcing the movement or rolling your head too quickly, as this can strain the muscles and joints.
- Breathe deeply and rhythmically as you perform the neck rolls, allowing the tension in your neck and shoulders to gradually release.

Time:

- Perform 5-10 repetitions of the Wall Neck Rolls in each direction, or as many as feels comfortable.
- Aim for smooth, controlled movement and focus on maintaining proper alignment throughout.

Benefits:

- Wall Neck Rolls help to improve flexibility and mobility in the neck, reducing stiffness and tension in the muscles.
- By gently stretching the muscles of the neck and shoulders, this exercise can help alleviate discomfort associated with tension headaches or neck strain.
- The rhythmic movement of the neck rolls can also promote relaxation and reduce stress, helping to improve overall well-being.

Tips:

- Focus on moving with awareness and control, paying attention to any areas of tension or discomfort in your neck and shoulders.
- If you experience any sharp pain or qdiscomfort during the neck rolls, stop the exercise immediately and consult with a healthcare professional.
- Incorporate Wall Neck Rolls into your daily routine to help improve neck mobility, reduce tension, and promote relaxation in the neck and shoulders.

Wall Ankle Circles

Starting Position:

- Stand facing a wall with your feet hip-width apart and arms relaxed by your sides.
- Place your hands lightly against the wall for support and stability.

Movement:

- Lift one foot off the ground and extend your leg forward slightly, keeping the knee straight.
- Begin to rotate your ankle in a circular motion, moving clockwise or counterclockwise.
- Perform the ankle circles slowly and with control, focusing on the range of motion in your ankle joint.
- After completing several circles in one direction, switch to the opposite direction to work the ankle from all angles.
- Repeat the movement with the other foot, alternating sides.

Positioning:

- Keep your standing leg slightly bent to maintain stability and prevent locking the knee joint.
- Engage your core muscles to stabilize your pelvis and maintain proper alignment throughout the exercise.

Execution:

- Move your ankle through its full range of motion, focusing on smooth and controlled movement.
- Avoid forcing the ankle into positions that cause pain or discomfort.
- Breathe deeply and rhythmically as you perform the ankle circles, maintaining a relaxed and steady breathing pattern.

Time:

- Perform 8-10 ankle circles in each direction for each foot, or as many as feels comfortable.
- Aim for smooth, controlled movement and focus on maintaining proper form throughout.

Benefits:

- Wall Ankle Circles help to improve mobility and flexibility in the ankle joint, reducing stiffness and tension in the muscles and ligaments.
- By moving the ankle through its full range of motion, this exercise can help improve proprioception and balance, reducing the risk of ankle injuries.
- The controlled movement of the ankle circles can also promote circulation and reduce swelling in the feet and ankles.

Tips:

- Focus on maintaining proper alignment and posture throughout the exercise, keeping your spine neutral and your shoulders relaxed.
- If you experience any discomfort or pain during the ankle circles, reduce the range of motion or stop the exercise altogether.
- Incorporate Wall Ankle Circles into your warm-up routine to prepare the ankles for more

strenuous activity, or use them as a gentle stretching exercise to relieve tension and promote flexibility in the ankles and feet.

COOL DOWN EXERCISE

Wall Supported Forward Fold

Starting Position:

- Stand facing a wall with your feet hip-width apart and arms relaxed by your sides.
- Take a step back with one foot and place it about one leg-length behind the other.
- Lean forward and place your palms flat against the wall at shoulder height.

Movement:

- Slowly begin to walk your hands down the wall, lowering your chest towards your thighs.
- Keep your back straight as you fold forward, hinging at your hips.
- Allow your head to relax and hang between your arms, releasing any tension in your neck and shoulders.
- Continue to walk your hands down the wall as far as feels comfortable, feeling a gentle stretch along the back of your legs and spine.
- Hold the stretched position for several breaths, focusing on relaxing into the stretch and letting go of any tension.

Positioning:

- Keep your feet firmly planted on the ground throughout the exercise, with your heels slightly lifted if necessary to maintain stability.
- Engage your core muscles to support your lower back and pelvis, preventing excessive arching or rounding of the spine.
- Relax your shoulders and allow your upper body to hang heavy as you fold forward.

Execution:

- Move slowly and with control, allowing your body to gradually sink deeper into the stretch.
- Focus on lengthening your spine and reaching your tailbone towards the wall behind you to deepen the stretch.
- Breathe deeply and rhythmically as you hold the forward fold, allowing each exhale to release tension and increase relaxation.

Time:

- Hold the Wall Supported Forward Fold for 30-60 seconds, or longer if you feel comfortable.

- Aim to relax into the stretch with each breath, allowing your body to soften and release tension.

Benefits:

- The Wall Supported Forward Fold helps to stretch the muscles of the hamstrings, lower back, and spine, reducing tension and promoting flexibility.
- By folding forward with support from the wall, this exercise allows you to relax into the stretch and release any gripping or holding patterns in the muscles.
- The gentle inversion provided by the forward fold can also help to calm the mind and reduce stress and anxiety.

Tips:

- Focus on maintaining a smooth and steady breath throughout the stretch, inhaling deeply to expand the ribcage and exhaling fully to release tension.
- If you experience any discomfort or pain during the forward fold, ease off slightly or adjust the position of your hands on the wall to reduce the intensity.
- Incorporate the Wall Supported Forward Fold into your cool-down routine to release tension in the muscles and promote relaxation and recovery after physical activity.

Wall-Assisted Downward-Facing Dog

Starting Position:

- Stand facing a wall with your feet hip-width apart and arms relaxed by your sides.
- Place your palms flat against the wall at shoulder height, with your fingers spread wide and pointing slightly upwards.
- Take a step back with one foot and then the other, until your body forms an inverted V-shape with your hips lifted towards the ceiling.

Movement:

- Press your palms firmly into the wall and straighten your arms, actively engaging your shoulders and upper back.
- Begin to walk your feet back towards the wall, allowing your heels to descend towards the floor.
- Keep your legs straight but not locked, with your heels reaching towards the ground and your toes pointing slightly inward.
- Lengthen your spine by lifting your hips higher towards the ceiling and pressing your chest towards your thighs.
- Hold the position for several breaths, feeling a stretch through your spine, hamstrings, calves, and shoulders.

Positioning:

- Keep your hands shoulder-width apart and shoulder-distance away from the wall, with your fingers spread wide for stability.
- Engage your core muscles to support your lower back and pelvis, preventing excessive arching or rounding of the spine.
- Press evenly through both hands and feet to distribute your weight evenly and avoid putting too much pressure on any one area.

Execution:

- Maintain a steady breath throughout the pose, inhaling deeply to expand the ribcage and exhaling fully to release tension.
- Focus on lengthening your spine and pressing your chest towards your thighs to deepen the stretch in your hamstrings and lower back.
- Keep your neck relaxed and gaze towards your feet or thighs, avoiding any strain or tension in the neck and shoulders.

Time:

- Hold the Wall-Assisted Downward-Facing Dog pose for 30-60 seconds, or longer if you feel comfortable.
- Aim to relax into the stretch with each breath, allowing your body to soften and release tension.

Benefits:

- The Wall-Assisted Downward-Facing Dog pose helps to stretch and lengthen the muscles of the spine, hamstrings, calves, shoulders, and arms.
- By using the wall for support, this variation of the pose allows you to focus on alignment and stability, making it accessible for practitioners of all levels.
- The inverted V-shape of the pose also helps to improve circulation and blood flow throughout the body, promoting relaxation and reducing stress.

Tips:

- Focus on maintaining a smooth and steady breath throughout the pose, inhaling deeply to expand the ribcage and exhaling fully to release tension.
- If you experience any discomfort or pain during the pose, ease off slightly or adjust the position of your hands or feet on the wall to reduce the intensity.
- Incorporate the Wall-Assisted Downward-Facing Dog pose into your cool-down routine to stretch and release tension in the muscles of the spine, hamstrings, calves, shoulders, and arms, promoting relaxation and recovery after physical activity.

Wall Side Bends

Starting Position:

- Stand upright with your side facing a wall, feet hip-width apart, and arms relaxed by your sides.
- Extend one arm overhead and place your palm flat against the wall, fingers pointing upwards.
- Keep your other arm relaxed by your side for balance.

Movement:

- Begin to lean sideways towards the wall, gently pressing your palm into the wall to support your upper body.
- Keep your feet planted firmly on the ground and your hips facing forward as you bend sideways.
- Feel a gentle stretch along the side of your torso, from your fingertips down to your hip.
- Hold the stretched position for several breaths, feeling the lengthening sensation along the side of your body.
- Slowly return to the starting position and repeat the movement on the opposite side.

Positioning:

- Maintain a neutral spine throughout the exercise, avoiding any excessive arching or rounding of the back.
- Keep your shoulders relaxed and away from your ears, avoiding any tension or shrugging.

- Engage your core muscles to support your spine and maintain stability.

Execution:

- Move slowly and with control, focusing on the sensation of the stretch along the side of your body.
- Avoid any jerky or abrupt movements, allowing your body to gradually ease into the stretch.
- Breathe deeply and rhythmically as you hold the side bend, allowing each exhale to deepen the stretch.

Time:

- Hold the Wall Side Bend for 20-30 seconds on each side, or longer if you feel comfortable.
- Aim for a total of 2-3 repetitions on each side, gradually increasing the duration of each stretch as your flexibility improves.

Benefits:

- Wall Side Bends help to stretch and lengthen the muscles along the side of the torso, including the obliques, intercostal muscles, and latissimus dorsi.
- By increasing flexibility and mobility in the side body, this exercise can improve overall posture and spinal alignment.
- The gentle stretching of the side body can also help to alleviate

tension and discomfort in the lower back and hips.

Tips:

- Focus on maintaining proper alignment and posture throughout the exercise, keeping your spine neutral and your shoulders relaxed.
- If you experience any discomfort or pain during the side bend, ease off slightly or adjust the intensity of the stretch.
- Incorporate Wall Side Bends into your regular stretching routine to improve flexibility and mobility in the side body, reduce tension, and promote better posture and spinal alignment.

Wall Supported Calf Raises

Starting Position:

- Stand upright with your back against a wall, feet hip-width apart, and arms relaxed by your sides.
- Keep your shoulders relaxed and your spine neutral, maintaining good posture throughout the exercise.

Movement:

- Place your palms flat against the wall at shoulder height for support.
- Slowly lift your heels off the ground, rising up onto the balls of your feet.
- Keep your ankles straight and your weight centered over the balls of your feet.
- Hold the raised position for a moment, feeling the contraction in your calf muscles.
- Lower your heels back down to the ground with control, returning to the starting position.
- Repeat the movement for the desired number of repetitions.

Positioning:

- Keep your feet parallel and hip-width apart throughout the exercise, with your toes pointing forward.
- Engage your core muscles to stabilize your spine and pelvis, preventing excessive arching or rounding of the back.
- Press evenly through both feet and keep your weight centered over the balls of your feet to maintain balance.

Execution:

- Move slowly and with control, focusing on the contraction and release of your calf muscle.
- Avoid any jerky or abrupt movements, maintaining smooth and controlled motion throughout.
- Breathe steadily throughout the exercise, inhaling as you lift your

heels and exhaling as you lower them back down.

Time:

- Perform 10-15 repetitions of Wall Supported Calf Raises, or as many as feels comfortable.
- Aim for 2-3 sets of calf raises, with a brief rest between sets to allow your muscles to recover.

Benefits:

- Wall Supported Calf Raises help to strengthen the calf muscles, including the gastrocnemius and soleus muscles, which are important for ankle stability and mobility.
- By strengthening the calf muscles, this exercise can help improve balance and reduce the risk of ankle injuries.
- The controlled motion of calf raises can also improve circulation in the lower legs and reduce the risk of muscle cramps and fatigue.

Tips:

- Focus on maintaining proper alignment and posture throughout the exercise, keeping your spine neutral and your shoulders relaxed.
- If you experience any discomfort or pain during calf raises, stop the exercise and consult with a healthcare professional.

- Gradually increase the number of repetitions and sets as your calf strength improves, but avoid overloading the muscles or pushing through pain.

Wall-Assisted Seated Piriformis Stretch

Starting Position:

- Sit on the floor with your back against a wall, legs extended in front of you.
- Bend your knees and bring the soles of your feet together, allowing your knees to fall out to the sides.
- Adjust your position so that your sitting bones are close to the wall and your spine is straight.

Movement:

- Gently lean back against the wall, using your hands for support as needed.
- Allow your knees to drop out to the sides, feeling a stretch in the outer hips and buttocks.
- Keep your spine tall and your chest lifted as you relax into the stretch.
- Hold the stretched position for 20-30 seconds, breathing deeply and allowing the tension to release.
- Slowly return to the starting position and repeat the stretch as desired.

Positioning:

- Keep your spine tall and your shoulders relaxed throughout the stretch.
- Engage your core muscles to support your lower back and pelvis, preventing excessive rounding or arching of the spine.
- Allow your knees to drop out to the sides naturally, without forcing them down.

Execution:

- Move gently and with control, focusing on the sensation of the stretch in the outer hips and buttocks.
- Avoid bouncing or jerking movements, as this can strain the muscles and joints.
- Breathe deeply and evenly as you hold the stretch, allowing each exhale to deepen the stretch.

Time:

- Hold the Wall-Assisted Seated Piriformis Stretch for 20-30 seconds on each side, or longer if you feel comfortable.
- Repeat the stretch 2-3 times on each side, gradually increasing the duration of each stretch as your flexibility improves.

Benefits:

- The Wall-Assisted Seated Piriformis Stretch targets the piriformis muscle, which can become tight and tense due to prolonged sitting or physical activity.
- By stretching the piriformis muscle, this exercise can help alleviate discomfort and improve flexibility in the hips and buttocks.
- The seated position against the wall provides support and stability, allowing you to relax into the stretch and release tension more effectively.

Tips:

- Focus on relaxing into the stretch and allowing the tension to release gradually.
- If you experience any discomfort or pain during the stretch, ease off slightly or adjust the intensity of the stretch.
- Incorporate the Wall-Assisted Seated Piriformis Stretch into your regular stretching routine to improve flexibility and mobility in the hips and buttocks, reduce tension, and alleviate discomfort associated with piriformis syndrome or tight hips.

Wall Supported Cat-Cow

Starting Position:

- Stand facing a wall with your feet hip-width apart and arms extended in front of you, palms flat against the wall at shoulder height.

- Engage your core muscles and maintain a neutral spine, with your shoulders relaxed and your gaze forward.

Movement:

- Inhale deeply and arch your back, pressing your chest forward and lifting your tailbone towards the ceiling.
- Allow your shoulder blades to come together behind you as you lift your chest.
- Exhale slowly and round your back, tucking your chin towards your chest and drawing your belly button towards your spine.
- Press your palms firmly into the wall as you round your back, feeling a stretch through your upper back and shoulders.
- Repeat the movement, flowing smoothly between the arching and rounding positions with each breath.

Positioning:

- Keep your feet firmly planted on the ground throughout the exercise, with your weight evenly distributed between both feet.
- Maintain a slight bend in your knees to prevent locking them and allow for fluid movement.
- Engage your core muscles to support your spine and pelvis, preventing excessive arching or rounding of the back.

Execution:

- Move slowly and with control, focusing on the sensation of the stretch in your spine and shoulders.
- Coordinate your breath with each movement, inhaling as you arch your back and exhaling as you round your back.
- Pay attention to the alignment of your spine and shoulders, keeping them in a straight line as you move through the Cat-Cow sequence.

Time:

- Flow through the Wall Supported Cat-Cow sequence for 1-2 minutes, allowing each breath to guide the movement.
- Focus on the quality of movement rather than the quantity of repetitions, aiming for smooth and controlled transitions between each position.

Benefits:

- The Wall Supported Cat-Cow helps to mobilize and stretch the spine, promoting flexibility and relieving tension in the back and shoulders.
- By coordinating movement with breath, this exercise can help

improve respiratory function and reduce stress and anxiety.
- The support of the wall provides stability and allows for deeper engagement of the core muscles, enhancing the effectiveness of the exercise.

Tips:

- Focus on moving with fluidity and grace, allowing each breath to guide the movement of your spine.
- Pay attention to any areas of tension or discomfort, and adjust the intensity of the stretch as needed.
- Incorporate the Wall Supported Cat-Cow into your regular stretching or warm-up routine to promote spinal mobility, relieve tension, and improve overall posture and alignment.

Deep Breaths

Deep breathing exercises are fundamental to the practice of Wall Pilates. These exercises, characterized by slow, deliberate breaths that fully expand the lungs and engage the diaphragm, play a pivotal role in promoting relaxation and mindfulness. As an integral aspect of Wall Pilates, understanding and mastering deep breathing techniques is essential for harnessing the full benefits of this exercise form.

Incorporating deep breathing into your Wall Pilates routine is not merely a suggestion but a necessity for achieving holistic well-being. Here's a breakdown of how deep breaths can enhance your Wall Pilates practice and overall sense of wellness:

Description: Deep breathing involves taking slow, deliberate breaths that fully engage the diaphragm and expand the lungs. These breaths are typically felt in the abdomen, rather than the chest, and are characterized by a sense of fullness and relaxation.

Technique: Start by finding a comfortable seated or standing position with your spine tall and shoulders relaxed. Inhale deeply through your nose, allowing your abdomen to expand fully. Feel the breath fill your lungs, gently lifting your chest. Exhale slowly and completely through your mouth, feeling your abdomen contract as you expel the air from your lungs. Repeat this process, focusing on the rhythm and depth of your breath.

Benefits: Deep breathing activates the body's relaxation response, reducing stress hormones and promoting a sense of calm. It increases oxygen intake and improves circulation, enhancing energy levels and mental clarity. Deep breathing can also alleviate symptoms of anxiety, depression, and other mood disorders by inducing relaxation and reducing physiological arousal.

Application in Wall Pilates: Incorporate deep breathing exercises at the beginning and end of your Wall Pilates sessions to center yourself and prepare for movement. Use deep breathing to enhance stretching exercises, promoting muscle relaxation and tension release. Practice deep breathing during challenging exercises to maintain focus and regulate your body's response to exertion.

Tips: Focus on breathing deeply into your abdomen, rather than shallow chest breathing. Take slow, controlled breaths, inhaling and exhaling at a comfortable pace. If your mind wanders during deep breathing exercises, gently redirect your focus back to your breath. Experiment with different techniques, such as counting breaths or incorporating pauses, to find what works best for you.

Deep breathing is not just a component of Wall Pilates; it's a cornerstone of the practice, essential for promoting relaxation, mindfulness, and overall well-being. Mastering the art of deep breathing will not only enhance your Wall Pilates experience but also enrich your life beyond the mat.

5

COMPREHENSIVE WALL PILATE EXERCISE

ABS AND CORE EXERCISE

Starting Position:

- Stand facing a wall with your feet hip-width apart.
- Place your palms flat against the wall at shoulder height, shoulder-width apart.
- Step back with one foot and then the other, until your body forms a straight line from head to heels.
- Engage your core muscles and maintain a neutral spine throughout the exercise.

Movement:

- Hold the Wall Plank position with your arms straight and palms pressing into the wall.
- Keep your body in a straight line from head to heels, avoiding any sagging or arching in the lower back.
- Focus on drawing your navel towards your spine to engage your deep core muscles.
- Breathe deeply and evenly as you hold the position, maintaining tension in your abdominal muscles.

Pose 1:

- In the starting position, ensure your wrists are aligned with your shoulders and your elbows are slightly bent.
- Keep your neck in line with your spine, avoiding any strain or tension.

Pose 2:

- As you hold the Wall Plank, focus on maintaining a strong, stable core.
- Engage your glutes and leg muscles to support your lower body and prevent sagging at the hips.
- Continue pressing your palms firmly into the wall to activate your chest and shoulder muscles.

Time:

- Hold the Wall Plank position for 20-30 seconds, gradually increasing the duration as you build strength and endurance.
- Aim for 2-3 sets of Wall Planks, with a brief rest between each set.

Tips:

- Focus on maintaining proper alignment and form throughout the exercise, keeping your body in a straight line from head to heels.
- If you feel any strain or discomfort in your lower back, adjust your position by slightly tilting your pelvis towards your ribs to engage your core muscles more effectively.

- Keep your breathing steady and controlled, inhaling deeply through your nose and exhaling fully through your mouth.
- If you're new to Wall Planks, start with shorter hold times and gradually increase the duration as you build strength and stability.
- Avoid holding your breath or allowing your shoulders to creep up towards your ears. Keep them relaxed and away from your neck.
- Remember to listen to your body and take breaks as needed. It's important to challenge yourself, but not at the expense of proper form and safety.

Modified Wall Plank

Starting Position:

- Stand facing a wall with your feet hip-width apart.
- Place your palms flat against the wall at shoulder height, slightly wider than shoulder-width apart.
- Step back with one foot and then the other, until your body forms a diagonal line from head to heels.
- Engage your core muscles and maintain a neutral spine throughout the exercise.

Movement:

- Hold the Modified Wall Plank position with your arms straight and palms pressing into the wall.
- Keep your body in a straight line from head to heels, avoiding any sagging or arching in the lower back.
- Focus on drawing your navel towards your spine to engage your deep core muscles.
- Breathe deeply and evenly as you hold the position, maintaining tension in your abdominal muscles.

Pose 1:

- Ensure your wrists are aligned with your shoulders and your elbows are slightly bent to reduce strain on the joints.
- Keep your neck in line with your spine, avoiding any strain or tension.

Pose 2:

- Maintain a strong, stable core throughout the Modified Wall Plank.
- Engage your glutes and leg muscles to support your lower body and prevent sagging at the hips.
- Continue pressing your palms firmly into the wall to activate your chest and shoulder muscles.

Time:

- Hold the Modified Wall Plank position for 20-30 seconds initially, gradually increasing the duration as you build strength and endurance.

- Aim for 2-3 sets of Modified Wall Planks, with a brief rest between each set.

Tips:

- Focus on maintaining proper alignment and form throughout the exercise, keeping your body in a straight line from head to heels.
- If you feel any strain or discomfort in your lower back, adjust your position by slightly tilting your pelvis towards your ribs to engage your core muscles more effectively.
- Keep your breathing steady and controlled, inhaling deeply through your nose and exhaling fully through your mouth.
- Start with shorter hold times and gradually increase the duration as you build strength and stability.
- Avoid holding your breath or allowing your shoulders to creep up towards your ears. Keep them relaxed and away from your neck.
- Listen to your body and take breaks as needed. It's important to challenge yourself, but not at the expense of proper form and safety.

Wall Knee Pulls

Starting Position:

- Stand facing a wall with your feet hip-width apart.
- Place your palms flat against the wall at shoulder height, shoulder-width apart.
- Engage your core muscles and maintain a neutral spine throughout the exercise.

Movement:

- Begin by lifting one knee towards your chest, bringing it as close to your torso as comfortably possible.
- Use your hands on the wall for support and stability as you bring the knee towards you.
- Keep your standing leg slightly bent to maintain balance and stability.
- Hold the position briefly, feeling the contraction in your abdominal muscles.
- Slowly return the lifted knee to the starting position and repeat the movement on the opposite side.

Pose:

- In the starting position, ensure your wrists are aligned with your shoulders and your elbows are slightly bent.
- Keep your neck in line with your spine, avoiding any strain or tension.

Time:

- Perform 10-15 repetitions of Wall

Knee Pulls on each leg, or as many as feels comfortable.

- Aim for 2-3 sets of knee pulls, with a brief rest between sets to allow your muscles to recover.

Tips:

- Focus on maintaining proper alignment and form throughout the exercise, keeping your body stable and avoiding excessive movement in your torso.
- Engage your core muscles to help stabilize your body as you lift and lower your knee.
- Keep your breathing steady and controlled throughout the movement, inhaling as you lift the knee and exhaling as you lower it.
- If you have any knee issues or discomfort, perform the movement with caution and avoid lifting the knee too high.
- Gradually increase the range of motion as you become more comfortable with the exercise, but always listen to your body and avoid pushing beyond your limits.

Wall Leg Lifts

Starting Position:

- Stand facing a wall with your feet hip-width apart.
- Place your palms flat against the wall at shoulder height, shoulder-width apart, for support.

- Engage your core muscles and maintain a neutral spine throughout the exercise.

Movement:

- Begin by lifting one leg straight out in front of you, keeping it parallel to the floor.
- Use the wall for support and stability as you lift the leg, pressing firmly into the wall with your hands.
- Keep your standing leg slightly bent to maintain balance and stability.
- Hold the lifted leg in position for a moment, feeling the engagement in your core and thigh muscles.
- Slowly lower the leg back down to the starting position and repeat the movement on the opposite side.

Pose:

- In the starting position, ensure your wrists are aligned with your shoulders and your elbows are slightly bent.
- Keep your neck in line with your spine, avoiding any strain or tension.

Time:

- Perform 10-15 repetitions of Wall Leg Lifts on each leg, or as many as feels comfortable.

- Aim for 2-3 sets of leg lifts, with a brief rest between sets to allow your muscles to recover.

Tips:

- Focus on maintaining proper alignment and form throughout the exercise, keeping your body stable and avoiding excessive movement in your torso.
- Engage your core muscles to help stabilize your body as you lift and lower your leg.
- Keep your breathing steady and controlled throughout the movement, inhaling as you lift the leg and exhaling as you lower it.
- If you have any knee issues or discomfort, perform the movement with caution and avoid lifting the leg too high.
- Gradually increase the range of motion as you become more comfortable with the exercise, but always listen to your body and avoid pushing beyond your limits.

Wall Side Plank

Starting Position:

- Stand sideways to a wall with your feet together.
- Place your forearm on the wall, elbow directly below your shoulder, forming a straight line from your shoulder to your wrist.
- Step your feet back away from the wall, stacking them on top of each other.
- Engage your core muscles and lift your hips so that your body forms a straight line from head to heels.

Movement:

- Hold the Wall Side Plank position, maintaining a straight line from your head to your heels.
- Keep your shoulder blades down and back, away from your ears, to avoid shrugging your shoulders.
- Focus on breathing deeply and evenly throughout the exercise, engaging your core muscles to maintain stability.
- Hold the position for the desired amount of time, ensuring proper form and alignment.

Pose:

- In the starting position, ensure your forearm is aligned with your shoulder, and your body forms a straight line from head to heels.
- Keep your neck in line with your spine, avoiding any strain or tension.

Time:

- Hold the Wall Side Plank position for 20-30 seconds on each side, gradually increasing the duration as you build strength and endurance.

- Aim for 2-3 sets of Wall Side Planks, with a brief rest between sets to allow your muscles to recover.

Tips:

- Focus on maintaining proper alignment and form throughout the exercise, keeping your body stable and avoiding any rotation or sagging at the hips.
- Engage your core muscles and squeeze your glutes to help stabilize your body in the plank position.
- Keep your breathing steady and controlled, inhaling deeply through your nose and exhaling fully through your mouth.
- If you experience any discomfort or strain, lower your bottom knee to the ground for added support or reduce the duration of the plank hold.
- As you become more comfortable with the exercise, challenge yourself by extending the duration of the hold or incorporating variations such as lifting the top leg or reaching the top arm towards the ceiling.

Modified Wall Side Plank

Starting Position:

- Stand sideways to a wall with your feet together.
- Place your forearm on the wall, elbow directly below your shoulder, forming a straight line from your shoulder to your wrist.
- Step your feet back away from the wall, stacking them on top of each other.
- Engage your core muscles and lift your hips so that your body forms a straight line from head to heels.

Movement:

- Hold the Modified Wall Side Plank position, maintaining a straight line from your head to your heels.
- Keep your shoulder blades down and back, away from your ears, to avoid shrugging your shoulders.
- Focus on breathing deeply and evenly throughout the exercise, engaging your core muscles to maintain stability.
- Hold the position for the desired amount of time, ensuring proper form and alignment.

Pose:

- In the starting position, ensure your forearm is aligned with your shoulder, and your body forms a straight line from head to heels.
- Keep your neck in line with your spine, avoiding any strain or tension.

Time:

- Hold the Modified Wall Side Plank position for 20-30 seconds on each side, gradually increasing

- the duration as you build strength and endurance.
- Aim for 2-3 sets of Modified Wall Side Planks, with a brief rest between sets to allow your muscles to recover.

Tips:

- Focus on maintaining proper alignment and form throughout the exercise, keeping your body stable and avoiding any rotation or sagging at the hips.
- Engage your core muscles and squeeze your glutes to help stabilize your body in the plank position.
- Keep your breathing steady and controlled, inhaling deeply through your nose and exhaling fully through your mouth.
- If you experience any discomfort or strain, lower your bottom knee to the ground for added support or reduce the duration of the plank hold.
- As you become more comfortable with the exercise, challenge yourself by extending the duration of the hold or incorporating variations such as lifting the top leg or reaching the top arm towards the ceiling.

Wall Bird Dog

Starting Position:

- Stand facing a wall with your feet hip-width apart.

- Place your palms flat against the wall at shoulder height, shoulder-width apart, for support.
- Engage your core muscles and maintain a neutral spine throughout the exercise.

Movement:

- Begin by lifting one arm straight out in front of you, parallel to the floor, while simultaneously lifting the opposite leg straight back behind you.
- Keep your hips level and avoid rotating your torso as you extend your arm and leg.
- Focus on reaching through your fingertips and toes to lengthen your body.
- Hold the extended position for a moment, feeling the engagement in your core muscles.
- Slowly lower your arm and leg back to the starting position and repeat the movement on the opposite side.

Pose:

- In the starting position, ensure your wrists are aligned with your shoulders and your elbows are slightly bent.
- Keep your neck in line with your spine, avoiding any strain or tension.

Time:

- Perform 10-15 repetitions of Wall

Bird Dogs on each side, or as many as feels comfortable.

- Aim for 2-3 sets of bird dogs, with a brief rest between sets to allow your muscles to recover.

Tips:

- Focus on maintaining proper alignment and form throughout the exercise, keeping your body stable and avoiding any arching or rounding of the back.
- Engage your core muscles to help stabilize your body as you lift and lower your arm and leg.
- Keep your breathing steady and controlled throughout the movement, inhaling as you extend your arm and leg and exhaling as you return to the starting position.
- If you have any shoulder or lower back issues, perform the movement with caution and avoid lifting the arm or leg too high.
- As you become more comfortable with the exercise, challenge yourself by increasing the range of motion or adding resistance with ankle weights.

Wall Cat-Cow with Modifications

Starting Position:

- Stand facing a wall with your feet hip-width apart.
- Place your palms flat against the wall at shoulder height, shoulder-width apart, for support.

- Engage your core muscles and maintain a neutral spine throughout the exercise.

Movement:

- Begin in a neutral spine position, with your back flat and your head in line with your spine.
- Inhale deeply and arch your back, allowing your belly to drop towards the floor and lifting your chest and tailbone towards the ceiling (Cow Pose).
- Exhale fully and round your back, tucking your chin towards your chest and drawing your belly button towards your spine (Cat Pose).
- Continue flowing between Cat and Cow Poses, moving with your breath and focusing on the movement of your spine.
- Use the wall for support and stability, pressing gently into it with your palms.

Pose:

- In the starting position, ensure your wrists are aligned with your shoulders and your elbows are slightly bent.
- Keep your neck in line with your spine, avoiding any strain or tension.

Time:

- Perform 8-10 repetitions of Wall

Cat-Cow, moving slowly and mindfully through each pose.

- Aim for 2-3 sets of Cat-Cow, with a brief rest between sets to allow your muscles to relax.

Modifications:

- If you have wrist issues or discomfort, perform Cat-Cow on your forearms instead of your palms. Place your forearms on the wall at shoulder height and perform the same spinal movements.
- If you have shoulder issues, perform Cat-Cow with your hands on a higher surface, such as a countertop or sturdy table, to reduce strain on your shoulders.
- If you have lower back issues, focus on moving gently and avoiding any excessive arching or rounding of the spine. Only move within a comfortable range of motion.

Tips:

- Focus on moving with your breath and maintaining a fluid, flowing motion between Cat and Cow Poses.
- Pay attention to how each movement feels in your body, and adjust the intensity or range of motion as needed.
- Keep your movements controlled and deliberate, avoiding any jerky or sudden movements that could strain your muscles or joints.

- Use the wall for support and stability throughout the exercise, pressing gently into it with your palms or forearms.
- Listen to your body and honor any sensations or limitations you experience during the exercise. If something doesn't feel right, back off or modify the movement accordingly.

Wall Hip Rolls

Starting Position:

- Stand facing a wall with your feet hip-width apart.
- Place your palms flat against the wall at shoulder height, shoulder-width apart, for support.
- Engage your core muscles and maintain a neutral spine throughout the exercise.

Movement:

- Begin by gently shifting your hips to one side, keeping your upper body facing forward.
- Initiate the movement from your hips, allowing them to roll towards the wall while keeping your feet firmly planted on the ground.
- Continue rolling your hips in a circular motion, moving from side to side and then forward and back.
- Use the wall for support and stability, pressing gently into it

with your palms as you move your hips.

- Focus on moving with control and fluidity, avoiding any jerky or abrupt movements.

Pose:

- In the starting position, ensure your wrists are aligned with your shoulders and your elbows are slightly bent.
- Keep your neck in line with your spine, avoiding any strain or tension.

Time:

- Perform 8-10 repetitions of Wall Hip Rolls in each direction, moving slowly and mindfully through each movement.
- Aim for 2-3 sets of Hip Rolls, with a brief rest between sets to allow your muscles to relax.

Tips:

- Focus on initiating the movement from your hips rather than your upper body, keeping your shoulders and chest facing forward.
- Keep your movements controlled and deliberate, avoiding any excessive twisting or strain on your lower back.
- Use your breath to help guide the movement, inhaling as you shift your hips one way and exhaling as you shift them the other way.

- Pay attention to how the movement feels in your body, and adjust the intensity or range of motion as needed.
- Use the wall for support and stability throughout the exercise, pressing gently into it with your palms to help maintain balance.

Wall Supported March

Starting Position:

- Stand facing a wall with your feet hip-width apart.
- Place your palms flat against the wall at shoulder height, shoulder-width apart, for support.
- Engage your core muscles and maintain a neutral spine throughout the exercise.

Movement:

- Begin by lifting one knee up towards your chest, bringing it as close to your torso as comfortably possible.
- Use the wall for support and stability, pressing gently into it with your palms as you lift your knee.
- Hold the lifted knee in position for a moment, feeling the engagement in your core and hip flexor muscles.
- Slowly lower the lifted knee back down to the ground and repeat the movement on the opposite side.

- Continue alternating between lifting each knee, moving in a controlled and deliberate manner.

Pose:

- In the starting position, ensure your wrists are aligned with your shoulders and your elbows are slightly bent.
- Keep your neck in line with your spine, avoiding any strain or tension.

Time:

- Perform 10-15 repetitions of Wall Supported March on each leg, or as many as feels comfortable.
- Aim for 2-3 sets of marches, with a brief rest between sets to allow your muscles to recover.

Tips:

- Focus on maintaining proper alignment and form throughout the exercise, keeping your body stable and avoiding any twisting or leaning to the side.
- Engage your core muscles to help stabilize your body as you lift and lower your knees.
- Keep your breathing steady and controlled throughout the movement, inhaling as you lift your knee and exhaling as you lower it.
- If you have any knee issues or discomfort, perform the

movement with caution and avoid lifting the knee too high.
- As you become more comfortable with the exercise, challenge yourself by increasing the speed or range of motion of the marches.

ARMS AND SHOULDER EXERCISE

Wall Arm Circles

Starting Position:

- Stand facing a wall with your feet hip-width apart.
- Extend your arms out to the sides, parallel to the floor, and place your palms flat against the wall.
- Engage your core muscles and maintain a neutral spine throughout the exercise.

Movement:

- Begin by making small circles with your arms, moving them forward in a circular motion.
- Use the wall for support and stability, pressing gently into it with your palms as you make the circles.
- Continue to increase the size of the circles, gradually moving your arms in larger rotations.
- Focus on maintaining control and stability in your shoulders and

core as you perform the movement.

- After completing several circles in the forward direction, reverse the motion and make circles with your arms moving backward.

Pose:

- In the starting position, ensure your wrists are aligned with your shoulders and your elbows are slightly bent.
- Keep your neck in line with your spine, avoiding any strain or tension.

Time:

- Perform 10-15 repetitions of Wall Arm Circles in each direction, or as many as feels comfortable.
- Aim for 2-3 sets of arm circles, with a brief rest between sets to allow your muscles to recover.

Tips:

- Focus on keeping your shoulders relaxed and down away from your ears throughout the movement.
- Engage your core muscles to help stabilize your body as you make the circles.
- Keep your breathing steady and controlled throughout the movement, inhaling as you circle your arms forward and exhaling as you circle them backward.
- If you have any shoulder issues or discomfort, perform the movement with caution and avoid excessive strain or range of motion.
- As you become more comfortable with the exercise, challenge yourself by increasing the speed or size of the circles.

Wall Diagonal Arm Raises

Starting Position:

- Stand facing a wall with your feet hip-width apart.
- Extend your arms out to the sides, parallel to the floor, and place your palms flat against the wall.
- Engage your core muscles and maintain a neutral spine throughout the exercise.

Movement:

- Begin by raising one arm diagonally upward and across your body towards these opposite corner of the wall.
- Keep your arm straight as you raise it, reaching towards the corner of the wall without rotating your torso.
- Use the wall for support and stability, pressing gently into it with your palm as you raise your arm.
- Pause briefly at the top of the movement, feeling the contraction in your shoulder muscles.

- Slowly lower your arm back down to the starting position and repeat the movement on the opposite side.

Pose:

- In the starting position, ensure your wrists are aligned with your shoulders and your elbows are slightly bent.
- Keep your neck in line with your spine, avoiding any strain or tension.

Time:

- Perform 10-15 repetitions of Wall Diagonal Arm Raises on each side, or as many as feels comfortable.
- Aim for 2-3 sets of arm raises, with a brief rest between sets to allow your muscles to recover.

Tips:

- Focus on maintaining proper alignment and form throughout the exercise, keeping your body stable and avoiding any twisting or leaning to the side.
- Engage your core muscles to help stabilize your body as you raise and lower your arms.
- Keep your breathing steady and controlled throughout the movement, inhaling as you raise your arm and exhaling as you lower it.

- If you have any shoulder issues or discomfort, perform the movement with caution and avoid lifting your arm too high.
- As you become more comfortable with the exercise, challenge yourself by increasing the speed or range of motion of the arm raises.

Wall Bicep Curls

Starting Position:

- Stand facing a wall with your feet hip-width apart.
- Extend your arms straight out in front of you, palms facing up, and place your palms flat against the wall.
- Engage your core muscles and maintain a neutral spine throughout the exercise.

Movement:

- Begin by bending your elbows and bringing your hands towards your shoulders, curling your fists towards your chest.
- Keep your upper arms stationary and close to your body throughout the movement.
- Use the wall for support and stability, pressing gently into it with your palms as you curl your fists.
- Pause briefly at the top of the movement, feeling the contraction in your bicep muscles.

- Slowly straighten your arms back out to the starting position and repeat the movement.

Pose:

- In the starting position, ensure your wrists are aligned with your shoulders and your elbows are slightly bent.
- Keep your neck in line with your spine, avoiding any strain or tension.

Time:

- Perform 10-15 repetitions of Wall Bicep Curls, or as many as feels comfortable.
- Aim for 2-3 sets of bicep curls, with a brief rest between sets to allow your muscles to recover.

Tips:

- Focus on keeping your elbows stationary and close to your body throughout the movement to maximize bicep engagement.
- Engage your core muscles to help stabilize your body as you perform the curls.
- Keep your breathing steady and controlled throughout the movement, inhaling as you curl your fists towards your chest and exhaling as you straighten your arms.
- If you have any wrist or elbow issues, perform the movement with caution and avoid using excessive weight.
- As you become more comfortable with the exercise, challenge yourself by increasing the resistance by using a resistance band or holding light weights in your hands.

Wall Tricep Extensions

Starting Position:

- Stand facing away from the wall with your feet hip-width apart.
- Extend your arms straight up overhead, palms facing forward, and place your palms flat against the wall.
- Engage your core muscles and maintain a neutral spine throughout the exercise.

Movement:

- Begin by bending your elbows and lowering your hands towards the wall behind you, keeping your upper arms close to your ears.
- Keep your elbows pointed forward and avoid letting them flare out to the sides.
- Use the wall for support and stability, pressing gently into it with your palms as you extend your arms.
- Pause briefly at the bottom of the movement, feeling the stretch in your tricep muscles.

- Slowly straighten your arms back up overhead to the starting position and repeat the movement.

Pose:

- In the starting position, ensure your wrists are aligned with your shoulders and your elbows are pointing forward.
- Keep your neck in line with your spine, avoiding any strain or tension.

Time:

- Perform 10-15 repetitions of Wall Tricep Extensions, or as many as feels comfortable.
- Aim for 2-3 sets of tricep extensions, with a brief rest between sets to allow your muscles to recover.

Tips:

- Focus on keeping your elbows close to your ears throughout the movement to maximize tricep engagement.
- Engage your core muscles to help stabilize your body as you perform the extensions.
- Keep your breathing steady and controlled throughout the movement, inhaling as you lower your hands towards the wall and exhaling as you extend your arms.
- If you have any shoulder or elbow issues, perform the movement with caution and avoid using excessive weight.
- As you become more comfortable with the exercise, challenge yourself by increasing the resistance by using a resistance band or holding light weights in your hands.

Wall Lateral Arm Raises

Starting Position:

- Stand facing a wall with your feet hip-width apart.
- Extend your arms straight out to the sides, parallel to the floor, and place your palms flat against the wall.
- Engage your core muscles and maintain a neutral spine throughout the exercise.

Movement:

- Begin by slowly raising both arms out to the sides until they are parallel to the floor.
- Keep your arms straight and your palms facing down as you lift them.
- Use the wall for support and stability, pressing gently into it with your palms as you raise your arms.
- Pause briefly at the top of the movement, feeling the contraction in your shoulder muscles.

- Slowly lower your arms back down to the starting position and repeat the movement.

Pose:

- In the starting position, ensure your wrists are aligned with your shoulders and your elbows are slightly bent.
- Keep your neck in line with your spine, avoiding any strain or tension.

Time:

- Perform 10-15 repetitions of Wall Lateral Arm Raises, or as many as feels comfortable.
- Aim for 2-3 sets of arm raises, with a brief rest between sets to allow your muscles to recover.

Tips:

- Focus on maintaining proper alignment and form throughout the exercise, keeping your body stable and avoiding any twisting or leaning to the side.
- Engage your core muscles to help stabilize your body as you raise and lower your arms.
- Keep your breathing steady and controlled throughout the movement, inhaling as you raise your arms and exhaling as you lower them.

- If you have any shoulder issues or discomfort, perform the movement with caution and avoid using excessive weight.
- As you become more comfortable with the exercise, challenge yourself by increasing the range of motion or adding resistance with light weights or resistance bands.

Wall Shoulder Rolls

Starting Position:

- Stand facing a wall with your feet hip-width apart.
- Keep your arms relaxed by your sides with your palms facing inward.

Movement:

- Begin by rolling your shoulders forward in a circular motion.
- Lift your shoulders up towards your ears, then roll them forward and down in a smooth, continuous motion.
- Use the wall for support and stability if needed, but allow your shoulders to move freely.
- After completing several forward rolls, reverse the motion and roll your shoulders backward in a circular motion.
- Lift your shoulders up towards your ears, then roll them backward and down in a smooth, continuous motion.

- Continue the backward rolls for several repetitions, focusing on loosening any tension in your shoulders.

Pose:

- Keep your neck relaxed and your chin parallel to the ground throughout the movement.
- Maintain a slight bend in your elbows to avoid locking them out.

Time:

- Perform 10-15 repetitions of Wall Shoulder Rolls in each direction, or as many as feels comfortable.
- Aim for 2-3 sets of shoulder rolls, with a brief rest between sets to allow your muscles to relax.

Tips:

- Focus on making the movement smooth and controlled, avoiding any jerky or sudden motions.
- Keep your breathing steady and relaxed throughout the exercise, inhaling as you lift your shoulders and exhaling as you lower them.
- Pay attention to any areas of tension or discomfort in your shoulders, and adjust the range of motion as needed to avoid strain.
- If you have any shoulder injuries or conditions, consult with a healthcare professional before performing this exercise to ensure it is safe for you.

- Incorporate Wall Shoulder Rolls into your warm-up routine to help increase blood flow to the shoulder muscles and improve mobility before more strenuous exercises.

Wall-Assisted Arm Raises

Starting Position:

- Stand facing a wall with your feet hip-width apart.
- Extend your arms out to the sides, parallel to the floor, and place your palms flat against the wall.
- Engage your core muscles and maintain a neutral spine throughout the exercise.

Movement:

- Begin by slowly raising one arm upward, keeping it straight as you lift it.
- Use the wall for support and stability, pressing gently into it with your palm as you raise your arm.
- Continue lifting your arm until it is overhead, or as high as you can comfortably reach.
- Pause briefly at the top of the movement, feeling the stretch in your shoulder muscles.
- Slowly lower your arm back down to the starting position and repeat the movement on the opposite side.

Pose:

- In the starting position, ensure your wrists are aligned with your shoulders and your elbows are slightly bent.
- Keep your neck in line with your spine, avoiding any strain or tension.

Time:

- Perform 10-15 repetitions of Wall-Assisted Arm Raises on each side, or as many as feels comfortable.
- Aim for 2-3 sets of arm raises, with a brief rest between sets to allow your muscles to recover.

Tips:

- Focus on maintaining proper alignment and form throughout the exercise, keeping your body stable and avoiding any twisting or leaning to the side.
- Engage your core muscles to help stabilize your body as you raise and lower your arms.
- Keep your breathing steady and controlled throughout the movement, inhaling as you raise your arm and exhaling as you lower it.
- If you have any shoulder issues or discomfort, perform the movement with caution and avoid using excessive weight.
- As you become more comfortable with the exercise, challenge yourself by increasing the range of motion or adding resistance with light weights or resistance bands.

LOWER BODY EXERCISE

Wall Squats

Starting Position:

- Stand with your back against a wall and your feet shoulder-width apart.
- Keep your feet about 1-2 feet away from the wall, depending on your flexibility and comfort.
- Engage your core muscles and maintain a neutral spine throughout the exercise.

Movement:

- Slowly slide your back down the wall, bending your knees and lowering your body into a squat position.
- Lower yourself until your thighs are parallel to the floor, or as close to parallel as you can comfortably go.
- Keep your knees aligned with your ankles and avoid letting them extend past your toes.
- Press your weight into your heels and keep your chest lifted throughout the movement.

- Hold the squat position for a few seconds, then push through your heels to return to the starting position.

Pose:

- Ensure your back remains flat against the wall throughout the exercise.
- Keep your neck in line with your spine, avoiding any strain or tension.

Time:

- Hold the squat position for 10-20 seconds, or as long as feels comfortable.
- Perform 8-12 repetitions of Wall Squats, or as many as feels challenging but manageable.
- Aim for 2-3 sets of squats, with a brief rest between sets to allow your muscles to recover.

Tips:

- Focus on keeping your knees aligned with your ankles and tracking in line with your toes to prevent strain on your joints.
- Engage your core muscles to help stabilize your body as you lower into and rise from the squat position.
- Keep your breathing steady and controlled throughout the movement, inhaling as you lower into the squat and exhaling as

you return to the starting position.
- If you have any knee issues or discomfort, perform the movement with caution and avoid lowering into a position that causes pain.
- As you become more comfortable with the exercise, challenge yourself by holding the squat position for longer durations or increasing the number of repetitions.

Modified Wall Squats

Starting Position:

- Stand facing a wall with your feet hip-width apart.
- Place your hands on the wall at shoulder height for support.
- Engage your core muscles and maintain a neutral spine throughout the exercise.

Movement:

- Slowly lower your body into a squat position by bending your knees and lowering your hips.
- Keep your knees aligned with your ankles and avoid letting them extend past your toes.
- Lower yourself as far as feels comfortable, aiming to bring your thighs parallel to the floor.
- Hold the squat position for a

moment, focusing on engaging your leg muscles.
- Push through your heels to return to the starting position, straightening your legs and rising back up.

Pose:

- Keep your back straight and your chest lifted throughout the movement.
- Ensure your knees stay aligned with your ankles and track in line with your toes.

Time:

- Hold the squat position for 5-10 seconds, or as long as feels comfortable.
- Perform 8-12 repetitions of Modified Wall Squats, or adjust the number based on your fitness level.
- Aim for 2-3 sets of squats, with a brief rest between sets to allow your muscles to recover.

Tips:

- Use the wall for support and stability, pressing gently into it with your hands as you lower into the squat.
- Focus on keeping your core engaged to help stabilize your body throughout the movement.
- Keep your breathing steady and controlled, inhaling as you lower into the squat and exhaling as you rise back up.
- If you have any knee issues or discomfort, adjust the depth of your squat to a level that feels comfortable for you.
- As you become more comfortable with the exercise, challenge yourself by holding the squat position for longer durations or increasing the number of repetitions.

Wall Calf Raises

Starting Position:

- Stand facing a wall with your feet hip-width apart.
- Place your hands on the wall at shoulder height for support.
- Engage your core muscles and maintain a neutral spine throughout the exercise.

Movement:

- Begin by lifting your heels off the ground, rising onto the balls of your feet.
- Keep your knees straight as you lift your heels, focusing on contracting your calf muscles.
- Lift your heels as high as you can comfortably go, feeling a stretch in your calf muscles.
- Hold the raised position for a moment, then lower your heels back down to the starting position.

- Repeat the movement, lifting and lowering your heels in a controlled manner.

Pose:

- Keep your back straight and your chest lifted throughout the movement.
- Ensure your knees stay aligned with your ankles and track in line with your toes.

Time:

- Perform 10-15 repetitions of Wall Calf Raises, or adjust the number based on your fitness level.
- Aim for 2-3 sets of calf raises, with a brief rest between sets to allow your muscles to recover.

Tips:

- Use the wall for support and stability, pressing gently into it with your hands as you perform the calf raises.
- Focus on lifting your heels as high as you can to fully engage your calf muscles.
- Keep your breathing steady and controlled, inhaling as you lift your heels and exhaling as you lower them.
- If you have any ankle issues or discomfort, perform the movement with caution and avoid lifting your heels too high.
- As you become more comfortable with the exercise, challenge yourself by increasing the number of repetitions or holding the raised position for longer durations.

Wall Single Leg Raises

Starting Position:

- Stand facing a wall with your feet hip-width apart.
- Place your hands on the wall at shoulder height for support.
- Engage your core muscles and maintain a neutral spine throughout the exercise.

Movement:

- Shift your weight onto one leg while keeping the other foot lightly touching the ground for balance.
- Slowly lift the non-weight-bearing foot off the ground, bringing your knee up towards your chest.
- Keep your standing leg slightly bent and your knee aligned with your ankle.
- Hold the raised position for a moment, feeling the engagement in your standing leg.
- Slowly lower your lifted leg back down to the ground with control.
- Repeat the movement on the opposite leg.

Pose:

- Keep your back straight and your chest lifted throughout the movement.
- Ensure your supporting knee stays aligned with your ankle and tracks in line with your toes.

Time:

- Perform 8-12 repetitions of Wall Single Leg Raises on each leg, or as many as feels challenging but manageable.
- Aim for 2-3 sets of single leg raises on each leg, with a brief rest between sets to allow your muscles to recover.

Tips:

- Use the wall for support and stability, pressing gently into it with your hands as you perform the single leg raises.
- Focus on keeping your core engaged to help stabilize your body throughout the movement.
- Keep your breathing steady and controlled, inhaling as you lift your leg and exhaling as you lower it.
- If you have any knee or ankle issues, perform the movement with caution and avoid lifting your leg too high.
- As you become more comfortable with the exercise, challenge yourself by increasing the number of repetitions or holding the raised position for longer durations.

Wall Side Leg Lifts

Starting Position:

- Stand sideways to a wall with your side facing the wall and your feet together.
- Place your hand on the wall for support at about hip or shoulder height.
- Engage your core muscles and maintain a neutral spine throughout the exercise.

Movement:

- Slowly lift your top leg directly out to the side, keeping it straight and parallel to the floor.
- Keep your foot flexed and your toes pointing forward as you lift your leg.
- Lift your leg as high as you can comfortably go, feeling the engagement in your hip and outer thigh muscles.
- Hold the raised position for a moment, focusing on maintaining balance and stability.
- Slowly lower your leg back down to the starting position with control.
- Repeat the movement for the desired number of repetitions on one side, then switch to the other side.

Pose:

- Keep your torso upright and your

shoulders relaxed throughout the movement.

- Ensure your supporting leg remains slightly bent to avoid locking the knee joint.

Time:

- Perform 10-15 repetitions of Wall Side Leg Lifts on each side, or adjust the number based on your fitness level.
- Aim for 2-3 sets of leg lifts on each side, with a brief rest between sets to allow your muscles to recover.

Tips:

- Use the wall for support and stability, pressing gently into it with your hand as you perform the leg lifts.
- Focus on keeping your core engaged to help stabilize your body throughout the movement.
- Keep your breathing steady and controlled, inhaling as you lift your leg and exhaling as you lower it.
- If you have any hip or knee issues, perform the movement with caution and avoid lifting your leg too high.
- As you become more comfortable with the exercise, challenge yourself by increasing the number of repetitions or adding ankle weights for added resistance.

Wall Hip Abduction

Starting Position:

- Stand sideways to a wall with your side facing the wall and your feet together.
- Place your hand on the wall for support at about hip or shoulder height.
- Engage your core muscles and maintain a neutral spine throughout the exercise.

Movement:

- Lift your top leg directly away from the wall, keeping it straight and parallel to the floor.
- Keep your foot flexed and your toes pointing forward as you lift your leg.
- Lift your leg as high as you can comfortably go, feeling the engagement in your hip and outer thigh muscles.
- Hold the raised position for a moment, focusing on maintaining balance and stability.
- Slowly lower your leg back down to the starting position with control.
- Repeat the movement for the desired number of repetitions on one side, then switch to the other side.

Pose:

- Keep your torso upright and your

shoulders relaxed throughout the movement.

- Ensure your supporting leg remains slightly bent to avoid locking the knee joint.

Time:

- Perform 10-15 repetitions of Wall Hip Abduction on each side, or adjust the number based on your fitness level.
- Aim for 2-3 sets of hip abductions on each side, with a brief rest between sets to allow your muscles to recover.

Tips:

- Use the wall for support and stability, pressing gently into it with your hand as you perform the hip abductions.
- Focus on keeping your core engaged to help stabilize your body throughout the movement.
- Keep your breathing steady and controlled, inhaling as you lift your leg and exhaling as you lower it.
- If you have any hip or knee issues, perform the movement with caution and avoid lifting your leg too high.
- As you become more comfortable with the exercise, challenge yourself by increasing the number of repetitions or adding ankle weights for added resistance.

Wall Heel Slides

Starting Position:

- Lie on your back with your legs extended and your feet flat against a wall.
- Keep your arms by your sides with your palms facing down for support.
- Engage your core muscles and maintain a neutral spine throughout the exercise.

Movement:

- Slide one heel down the wall, bending your knee and bringing your foot towards your buttocks.
- Keep the other leg extended and pressed against the wall throughout the movement.
- Slide your heel as far down the wall as you can comfortably go, feeling the stretch in your quadriceps.
- Hold the stretched position for a moment, focusing on maintaining tension in the muscle.
- Slowly return your heel back up the wall to the starting position with control.
- Repeat the movement on the opposite leg.

Pose:

- Keep your hips and pelvis stable throughout the movement, avoiding any rocking or tilting.

- Ensure your shoulders remain relaxed on the floor.

Time:

- Perform 8-12 repetitions of Wall Heel Slides on each leg, or as many as feels challenging but manageable.
- Aim for 2-3 sets of heel slides on each leg, with a brief rest between sets to allow your muscles to recover.

Tips:

- Focus on keeping your core engaged to help stabilize your body throughout the movement.
- Keep your breathing steady and controlled, inhaling as you slide your heel down the wall and exhaling as you return it to the starting position.
- If you experience any discomfort in your knees or hips, perform the movement with caution and avoid sliding your heel too far down the wall.
- As you become more comfortable with the exercise, challenge yourself by increasing the range of motion or holding the stretched position for longer durations.

Modified Wall Piriformis Stretch

Starting Position:

- Lie on your back with your knees bent and your feet flat on the floor.
- Extend your arms out to the sides with your palms facing down for support.
- Engage your core muscles and maintain a neutral spine throughout the exercise.

Movement:

- Cross your right ankle over your left knee, creating a figure-four shape with your legs.
- Keep your right foot flexed to protect your knee and ankle joints.
- Gently press your right knee away from your body, feeling the stretch in your right hip and buttocks.
- Hold the stretch for 15-30 seconds, focusing on relaxing into the sensation.
- Slowly release the stretch and switch legs, crossing your left ankle over your right knee.
- Repeat the stretch on the opposite side.

Pose:

- Keep your shoulders and hips flat on the floor throughout the stretch.
- Ensure your neck remains relaxed, avoiding any tension in the muscles.

Time:

- Hold each stretch for 15-30 seconds, or as long as feels comfortable.
- Repeat the stretch 2-3 times on each side, gradually increasing the duration of the hold with each repetition.

Tips:

- Focus on breathing deeply and evenly throughout the stretch, inhaling through your nose and exhaling through your mouth.
- Adjust the intensity of the stretch by gently pressing your knee away from your body or bringing it closer, depending on your flexibility and comfort level.
- If you experience any discomfort or pain during the stretch, ease off the pressure and adjust your positioning as needed.
- Incorporate the Modified Wall Piriformis Stretch into your regular stretching routine to help improve hip mobility and reduce tension in the buttocks and lower back.
- Consult with a healthcare professional if you have any pre-existing hip or lower back conditions before performing this stretch, to ensure it is safe for you.

Wall-Assisted Downward-Facing Dog

Starting Position:

- Stand facing a wall with your feet hip-width apart.
- Place your hands on the wall at about shoulder height, shoulder-width apart.
- Walk your feet back until your body forms an inverted V shape, with your hips lifted toward the ceiling.

Movement:

- Press your palms firmly into the wall and straighten your arms, creating a straight line from your wrists to your hips.
- Engage your core muscles and lengthen your spine, allowing your head to hang between your arms.
- Press your heels down toward the floor to feel a stretch in your calves and hamstrings.
- Hold the position for 15-30 seconds, breathing deeply and evenly.
- To release, walk your feet back toward the wall and return to a standing position.

Pose:

- Keep your shoulders relaxed and away from your ears, allowing your neck to lengthen.

- Keep your knees slightly bent if you feel any strain in your hamstrings or lower back.

Time:

- Hold the Wall-Assisted Downward-Facing Dog pose for 15-30 seconds, or as long as feels comfortable.
- Repeat the pose 2-3 times, with a brief rest between repetitions.

Tips:

- Focus on pressing your palms firmly into the wall to create a stable foundation for the pose.
- Lengthen your spine by reaching your tailbone toward the ceiling and drawing your ribs in toward your spine.
- Keep your gaze directed toward your feet or your navel to maintain alignment in the pose.
- If you feel any discomfort in your wrists, try spreading your fingers wide and distributing your weight evenly through your palms.
- Use the Wall-Assisted Downward-Facing Dog pose as a gentle stretch for your calves, hamstrings, shoulders, and back, or as part of a longer yoga practice to build strength and flexibility.

FLEXIBLE AND BALANCE EXERCISE

Wall Hamstring Stretch

Starting Position:

- Lie on your back with your legs extended and your buttocks close to a wall.
- Place your arms by your sides with your palms facing down for support.

Movement:

- Lift your legs up and extend them against the wall, forming a 90-degree angle with your body.
- Flex your feet and press them gently against the wall, feeling a stretch in the back of your legs.
- Keep your legs straight and your knees soft, avoiding any locking of the knee joints.
- Relax into the stretch and hold the position for 30-60 seconds, breathing deeply and evenly.
- To release, bend your knees and slide your feet down the wall until your heels touch the floor.
- Repeat the stretch for 2-3 sets, gradually increasing the duration of the hold with each repetition.

Pose:

- Keep your shoulders and hips flat on the floor throughout the stretch.

- Maintain a neutral spine and avoid arching your lower back excessively.

Time:

- Hold the Wall Hamstring Stretch for 30-60 seconds, or as long as feels comfortable.
- Repeat the stretch for 2-3 sets, with a brief rest between sets to allow your muscles to recover.

Tips:

- Focus on relaxing into the stretch and allowing your muscles to release tension gradually.
- Keep your breathing steady and controlled, inhaling deeply through your nose and exhaling fully through your mouth.
- If you feel any discomfort or pain during the stretch, ease off the intensity and adjust your positioning as needed.
- Use the Wall Hamstring Stretch as part of a comprehensive flexibility routine to improve mobility in your hamstrings and lower back.
- Consult with a healthcare professional if you have any pre-existing conditions or injuries that may affect your ability to perform this stretch safely.

Wall Side Bends

Starting Position:

- Stand with your side facing a wall, feet hip-width apart, and arms relaxed by your sides.
- Ensure your feet are positioned about a foot away from the wall.

Movement:

- Inhale deeply, lengthening your spine and engaging your core muscles.
- As you exhale, slowly lean sideways towards the wall, keeping your body in a straight line.
- Place your hand on the wall for support as you bend, allowing your other arm to extend overhead.
- Feel a gentle stretch along the side of your body from your fingertips to your hip.
- Hold the stretch for 15-30 seconds, breathing deeply and maintaining stability.
- Inhale as you return to the starting position, engaging your core to lift back up.
- Repeat the movement on the opposite side, bending towards the other side of the wall.

Pose:

- Keep your shoulders relaxed and away from your ears throughout the movement.

- Ensure your hips remain aligned and facing forward, avoiding any twisting or rotation.

Time:

- Hold each Wall Side Bend for 15-30 seconds, or as long as feels comfortable.
- Repeat the stretch 2-3 times on each side, gradually increasing the duration of the hold with each repetition.

Tips:

- Focus on maintaining stability and control throughout the movement, avoiding any sudden or jerky motions.
- Keep your breathing steady and controlled, inhaling deeply as you prepare to bend and exhaling slowly as you lean into the stretch.
- Adjust the intensity of the stretch by moving your hand higher or lower on the wall, depending on your flexibility and comfort level.
- Use the Wall Side Bends as a gentle way to improve flexibility in your side body and increase mobility in your spine.
- Incorporate this exercise into your warm-up routine or as part of a larger flexibility regimen to enhance overall range of motion.

Wall Piriformis Stretch

Starting Position:

- Lie on your back with your knees bent and your feet flat on the floor.
- Extend your arms out to the sides with your palms facing down for support.
- Engage your core muscles and maintain a neutral spine throughout the exercise.

Movement:

- Cross your right ankle over your left knee, creating a figure-four shape with your legs.
- Keep your right foot flexed to protect your knee and ankle joints.
- Gently press your right knee away from your body, feeling the stretch in your right hip and buttocks.
- Hold the stretch for 15-30 seconds, focusing on relaxing into the sensation.
- Slowly release the stretch and switch legs, crossing your left ankle over your right knee.
- Repeat the stretch on the opposite side.

Pose:

- Keep your shoulders and hips flat on the floor throughout the stretch.
- Ensure your neck remains relaxed, avoiding any tension in the muscles.

Time:

- Hold each stretch for 15-30 seconds, or as long as feels comfortable.
- Repeat the stretch 2-3 times on each side, gradually increasing the duration of the hold with each repetition.

Tips:

- Focus on breathing deeply and evenly throughout the stretch, inhaling through your nose and exhaling through your mouth.
- Adjust the intensity of the stretch by gently pressing your knee away from your body or bringing it closer, depending on your flexibility and comfort level.
- If you experience any discomfort or pain during the stretch, ease off the pressure and adjust your positioning as needed.
- Incorporate the Wall Piriformis Stretch into your regular stretching routine to help improve hip mobility and reduce tension in the buttocks and lower back.
- Consult with a healthcare professional if you have any pre-existing hip or lower back conditions before performing this stretch, to ensure it is safe for you.

Wall Cat-Cow

Starting Position:

- Stand facing a wall with your feet hip-width apart.
- Place your hands on the wall at about shoulder height, shoulder-width apart.
- Keep your arms straight and your fingers spread wide for stability.

Movement:

- Inhale deeply as you arch your back, lowering your chest towards the wall and lifting your tailbone upwards (Cow Pose).
- Allow your shoulder blades to come together and your chest to open.
- Exhale as you round your spine, pushing your hands into the wall and tucking your chin towards your chest (Cat Pose).
- Draw your belly button towards your spine to deepen the stretch in your back.
- Flow smoothly between Cat and Cow poses, coordinating your breath with each movement.
- Repeat the sequence for 8-10 repetitions, moving at a pace that feels comfortable.

Pose:

- Keep your arms straight and your shoulders relaxed throughout the movement.
- Engage your core muscles to support your spine and maintain stability.

Time:

- Perform 8-10 repetitions of the Wall Cat-Cow exercise, moving with your breath.
- Focus on the quality of movement rather than the quantity of repetitions.

Tips:

- Move slowly and mindfully, paying attention to how each movement feels in your body.
- Coordinate your breath with the movement to enhance relaxation and improve flexibility.
- Focus on elongating your spine in Cow Pose and rounding your back in Cat Pose to maximize the stretch.
- Use the Wall Cat-Cow exercise as a gentle warm-up or cooldown for your spine and core muscles.
- If you experience any discomfort or pain, adjust the range of motion or consult with a healthcare professional.

Wall Ankle Circles

Starting Position:

- Stand facing a wall with your feet hip-width apart.
- Place your hands on the wall for support at about shoulder height.

Movement:

- Lift one foot off the ground and extend it forward.
- Rotate your ankle in a circular motion, starting with small circles and gradually increasing the size.
- Perform 8-10 circles in one direction, then reverse and perform 8-10 circles in the opposite direction.
- Keep your movements controlled and fluid, focusing on the range of motion in your ankle joint.
- Switch to the other foot and repeat the exercise.

Pose:

- Keep your standing leg slightly bent to maintain stability.
- Maintain good posture with your shoulders relaxed and your core engaged.

Time:

- Perform 8-10 ankle circles in each direction on each foot.
- Aim for 2-3 sets of ankle circles on each foot, with a brief rest between sets.

Tips:

- Focus on drawing full circles with your ankle, exploring the entire range of motion.
- Keep your movements slow and deliberate to avoid straining the ankle joint.

- If you experience any discomfort or pain, reduce the size of the circles or stop the exercise.
- Use the Wall Ankle Circles as part of your warm-up routine to increase blood flow and flexibility in the ankles.
- Incorporate ankle circles into your daily routine to improve ankle mobility and prevent stiffness.

Wall Single Leg Stands

Starting Position:

- Stand facing a wall with your feet hip-width apart.
- Place your hands lightly on the wall for support at about shoulder height.

Movement:

- Lift one foot off the ground and balance on the other foot.
- Keep your lifted foot slightly off the floor, either hovering just above or lightly touching the ground for balance.
- Engage your core muscles to stabilize your body and maintain good posture.
- Hold the single-leg stance for 15-30 seconds, focusing on your balance and stability.
- If you feel comfortable, challenge yourself by closing your eyes or lifting your arms away from the wall for an additional balance challenge.
- Switch to the other foot and repeat the exercise.

Pose:

- Keep your standing leg slightly bent to absorb any slight movements and maintain balance.
- Maintain a neutral spine with your shoulders relaxed and your chest lifted.

Time:

- Hold the single-leg stance for 15-30 seconds on each foot.
- Aim for 2-3 sets of single-leg stands on each foot, with a brief rest between sets.

Tips:

- Focus on a fixed point on the wall to help maintain your balance.
- Engage your core muscles and imagine a string pulling you up from the top of your head to help stabilize your body.
- Start with shorter holds and gradually increase the duration as your balance improves.
- If you struggle with balance, practice near a stable surface like a countertop or chair before attempting the wall single-leg stand.
- Use the wall single-leg stand to improve your balance and

strengthen stabilizing muscles in your legs and core.

Wall Heel-Toe Walk

Starting Position:

- Stand facing a wall with your feet hip-width apart.
- Place your hands lightly on the wall for support at about shoulder height.

Movement:

- Lift your heels off the ground, balancing on the balls of your feet.
- Slowly walk forward, placing one foot directly in front of the other so that the heel of each foot touches the toes of the opposite foot.
- Maintain a smooth and controlled movement, focusing on the alignment of your feet and ankles.
- Continue walking for a few steps, keeping your gaze forward and your core engaged.
- Reverse the movement by walking backward in the same heel-to-toe pattern.
- Repeat the forward and backward walks for several repetitions.

Pose:

- Keep your shoulders relaxed and your chest lifted throughout the exercise.

- Maintain a neutral spine and engage your core muscles to stabilize your body.

Time:

- Perform the heel-toe walk for 10-15 steps forward and backward, or as far as space allows.
- Aim for 2-3 sets of heel-toe walks, with a brief rest between sets.

Tips:

- Focus on placing each foot deliberately and maintaining balance throughout the movement.
- Keep your movements slow and controlled to maximize the balance challenge.
- Use the wall for support as needed, but try to rely on your own balance as much as possible.
- Practice the heel-toe walk regularly to improve balance, ankle stability, and proprioception.
- Gradually increase the difficulty by walking on a narrow line or uneven surface once you feel comfortable with the basic heel-toe walk.

6

SPECIALIZES WORKOUT PROGRAM

Warm up Routine (10 min)

Day 1: Monday - Wall Pilates Warm-Up

Wall Hamstrings Stretch (2 minutes)
Wall Cat-Cow (2 minutes)
Wall Lateral Arm Raises (2 minutes)
Wall Chest Openers (2 minutes)
Wall Ankle Circles (2 minutes)

Day 2: Tuesday - Wall Pilates Warm-Up

Wall Heel Slides (2 minutes)
Wall Arm Circles (2 minutes)
Wall Leg Lifts (2 minutes)
Wall Piriformis Stretch (2 minutes)
Wall Neck Rolls (2 minutes)

Day 3: Wednesday - Wall Pilates Warm-Up

Wall Hamstrings Stretch (2 minutes)
Wall Lateral Arm Raises (2 minutes)
Wall Chest Openers (2 minutes)
Wall Ankle Circles (2 minutes)
Wall Cat-Cow (2 minutes)

Day 4: Thursday - Wall Pilates Warm-Up

Wall Leg Lifts (2 minutes)
Wall Piriformis Stretch (2 minutes)
Wall Neck Rolls (2 minutes)
Wall Heel Slides (2 minutes)
Wall Arm Circles (2 minutes)

Day 5: Friday - Wall Pilates Warm-Up

Wall Chest Openers (2 minutes)
Wall Ankle Circles (2 minutes)
Wall Cat-Cow (2 minutes)
Wall Lateral Arm Raises (2 minutes)
Wall Hamstrings Stretch (2 minutes)

Day 6: Saturday - Wall Pilates Warm-Up

Wall Piriformis Stretch (2 minutes)
Wall Neck Rolls (2 minutes)
Wall Heel Slides (2 minutes)
Wall Arm Circles (2 minutes)
Wall Leg Lifts (2 minutes)
Day 7: Sunday - Rest Day

Day 8: Monday - Wall Pilates Warm-Up

Wall Leg Lifts (2 minutes)
Wall Hamstrings Stretch (2 minutes)
Wall Heel Slides (2 minutes)
Wall Arm Circles (2 minutes)
Wall Chest Openers (2 minutes)

Day 9: Tuesday - Wall Pilates Warm-Up

Wall Piriformis Stretch (2 minutes)
Wall Neck Rolls (2 minutes)
Wall Lateral Arm Raises (2 minutes)
Wall Cat-Cow (2 minutes)
Wall Ankle Circles (2 minutes)

Day 10: Wednesday - Wall Pilates Warm-Up

Wall Cat-Cow (2 minutes)
Wall Hamstrings Stretch (2 minutes)
Wall Arm Circles (2 minutes)
Wall Heel Slides (2 minutes)
Wall Leg Lifts (2 minutes)

Day 11: Thursday - Wall Pilates Warm-Up

Wall Chest Openers (2 minutes)
Wall Piriformis Stretch (2 minutes)
Wall Ankle Circles (2 minutes)
Wall Neck Rolls (2 minutes)
Wall Lateral Arm Raises (2 minutes)

Day 12: Friday - Wall Pilates Warm-Up

Wall Heel Slides (2 minutes)
Wall Leg Lifts (2 minutes)
Wall Cat-Cow (2 minutes)
Wall Hamstrings Stretch (2 minutes)
Wall Arm Circles (2 minutes)

Day 13: Saturday - Wall Pilates Warm-Up

Wall Arm Circles (2 minutes)
Wall Chest Openers (2 minutes)
Wall Lateral Arm Raises (2 minutes)
Wall Ankle Circles (2 minutes)
Wall Piriformis Stretch (2 minutes)

Day 14: Sunday - Rest Day

Cooldown Routine

Day 1: Wall Pilates Cool-Down

Wall Supported Forward Fold (2 minutes)
Wall-Assisted Downward-Facing Dog (2 minutes)
Wall Side Bends (2 minutes)
Wall Supported Calf Raises (2 minutes)
Wall-Assisted Seated Piriformis Stretch (2 minutes)

Day 2: Wall Pilates Cool-Down

Wall Supported Cat-Cow (2 minutes)
Deep Breaths (2 minutes)
Wall Side Bends (2 minutes)
Wall-Assisted Seated Piriformis Stretch (2 minutes)
Wall Supported Forward Fold (2 minutes)

Day 3: Wall Pilates Cool-Down

Wall-Assisted Downward-Facing Dog (2 minutes)
Wall Supported Calf Raises (2 minutes)
Deep Breaths (2 minutes)
Wall Supported Forward Fold (2 minutes)
Wall Side Bends (2 minutes)

Day 4: Wall Pilates Cool-Down

Wall Supported Calf Raises (2 minutes)
Wall-Assisted Seated Piriformis Stretch (2 minutes)

Deep Breaths (2 minutes)
Wall Side Bends (2 minutes)
Wall Supported Cat-Cow (2 minutes)

Day 5: Wall Pilates Cool-Down

Deep Breaths (2 minutes)
Wall Supported Forward Fold (2 minutes)
Wall-Assisted Downward-Facing Dog (2 minutes)
Wall Supported Cat-Cow (2 minutes)
Wall Side Bends (2 minutes)

Day 6: Wall Pilates Cool-Down

Wall Supported Calf Raises (2 minutes)
Wall-Assisted Seated Piriformis Stretch (2 minutes)
Deep Breaths (2 minutes)
Wall Side Bends (2 minutes)
Wall Supported Forward Fold (2 minutes)

Day 7: Wall Pilates Cool-Down

Rest Day

Day 8: Wall Pilates Cool-Down

Wall Side Bends (2 minutes)
Wall Supported Cat-Cow (2 minutes)
Deep Breaths (2 minutes)
Wall Supported Forward Fold (2 minutes)

Day 9: Wall Pilates Cool-Down

Wall Supported Forward Fold (2 minutes)
Deep Breaths (2 minutes)
Wall-Assisted Downward-Facing Dog (2 minutes)
Wall Side Bends (2 minutes)
Wall Supported Calf Raises (2 minutes)

Day 10: Wall Pilates Cool-Down

Wall-Assisted Seated Piriformis Stretch (2 minutes)
Wall Supported Calf Raises (2 minutes)
Wall Side Bends (2 minutes)
Deep Breaths (2 minutes)
Wall Supported Cat-Cow (2 minutes)

Day 11: Wall Pilates Cool-Down

Wall Supported Forward Fold (2 minutes)
Wall-Assisted Downward-Facing Dog (2 minutes)
Deep Breaths (2 minutes)
Wall Supported Cat-Cow (2 minutes)
Wall Side Bends (2 minutes)

Day 12: Wall Pilates Cool-Down

Deep Breaths (2 minutes)

Wall Supported Forward Fold (2 minutes)
Wall Side Bends (2 minutes)
Wall-Assisted Seated Piriformis Stretch (2 minutes)
Wall Supported Calf Raises (2 minutes)

Day 13: Wall Pilates Cool-Down

Wall Supported Cat-Cow (2 minutes)
Wall-Assisted Downward-Facing Dog (2 minutes)
Wall Supported Forward Fold (2 minutes)
Wall Side Bends (2 minutes)
Deep Breaths (2 minutes)

Day 14: Wall Pilates Cool-Down

Rest Day

Flexibility Focus Weekly Workout Plan

Week 1

Day 1: Flexibility and Core

- **Warm-Up:** Wall Hamstrings Stretch, Wall Cat-Cow, Wall Arm Circles
- **ABS and Core Exercise:** Wall Plank, Modified Wall Plank, Wall Knee Pulls
- **Cool-Down:** Wall Supported Forward Fold, Wall-Assisted Downward-Facing Dog, Wall Side Bends

Day 2: Arms and Shoulders

- **Warm-Up:** Wall Heel Slides, Wall Lateral Arm Raises, Wall Chest Openers
- **Arms and Shoulder Exercise:** Wall Arm Circles, Wall Diagonal Arm Raises, Wall Bicep Curls
- **Cool-Down:** Wall Supported Calf Raises, Wall-Assisted Seated Piriformis Stretch, Wall Supported Cat-Cow

Day 3: Lower Body

- **Warm-Up:** Wall Leg Lifts, Wall Piriformis Stretch, Wall Neck Rolls
- **Lower Body Exercise:** Wall Squats, Modified Wall Squats, Wall Calf Raises
- **Cool-Down:** Wall Single Leg Raises, Wall Side Leg Lifts, Wall Hip Abduction

Day 4: Flexibility and Balance

- **Warm-Up:** Wall Hamstrings Stretch, Wall Side Bends, Wall Piriformis Stretch
- **Flexibility and Balance Exercise:** Wall Ankle Circles, Wall Single Leg Stands, Wall Heel-Toe Walk

- **Cool-Down:** Wall Cat-Cow, Deep Breaths

Day 5: Flexibility and Core

- **Warm-Up:** Wall Hamstrings Stretch, Wall Cat-Cow, Wall Arm Circles
- **ABS and Core Exercise:** Wall Plank, Modified Wall Plank, Wall Knee Pulls
- **Cool-Down:** Wall Supported Forward Fold, Wall-Assisted Downward-Facing Dog, Wall Side Bends

Day 6: Arms and Shoulders

- **Warm-Up:** Wall Heel Slides, Wall Lateral Arm Raises, Wall Chest Openers
- **Arms and Shoulder Exercise:** Wall Arm Circles, Wall Diagonal Arm Raises, Wall Bicep Curls
- **Cool-Down:** Wall Supported Calf Raises, Wall-Assisted Seated Piriformis Stretch, Wall Supported Cat-Cow

Day 7: Rest Day

Week 2

Day 1: Flexibility and Core

- **Warm-Up:** Wall Hamstrings Stretch, Wall Cat-Cow, Wall Arm Circles

- **ABS and Core Exercise:** Wall Plank, Modified Wall Plank, Wall Knee Pulls
- **Cool-Down:** Wall Supported Forward Fold, Wall-Assisted Downward-Facing Dog, Wall Side Bends

Day 2: Arms and Shoulders

- **Warm-Up:** Wall Heel Slides, Wall Lateral Arm Raises, Wall Chest Openers
- **Arms and Shoulder Exercise:** Wall Arm Circles, Wall Diagonal Arm Raises, Wall Bicep Curls
- **Cool-Down:** Wall Supported Calf Raises, Wall-Assisted Seated Piriformis Stretch, Wall Supported Cat-Cow

Day 3: Lower Body

- **Warm-Up:** Wall Leg Lifts, Wall Piriformis Stretch, Wall Neck Rolls
- **Lower Body Exercise:** Wall Squats, Modified Wall Squats, Wall Calf Raises
- **Cool-Down:** Wall Single Leg Raises, Wall Side Leg Lifts, Wall Hip Abduction

Day 4: Flexibility and Balance

- **Warm-Up:** Wall Hamstrings Stretch, Wall Side Bends, Wall Piriformis Stretch
- **Flexibility and Balance Exercise:** Wall Ankle Circles,

Wall Single Leg Stands, Wall
Heel-Toe Walk
- **Cool-Down:** Wall Cat-Cow,
Deep Breaths

Day 5: Flexibility and Core

- **Warm-Up:** Wall Hamstrings
Stretch, Wall Cat-Cow, Wall Arm
Circles
- **ABS and Core Exercise:** Wall
Plank, Modified Wall Plank, Wall
Knee Pulls
- **Cool-Down:** Wall Supported
Forward Fold, Wall-Assisted
Downward-Facing Dog, Wall Side
Bends

Day 6: Arms and Shoulders

- **Warm-Up:** Wall Heel Slides,
Wall Lateral Arm Raises, Wall
Chest Openers
- **Arms and Shoulder Exercise:**
Wall Arm Circles, Wall Diagonal
Arm Raises, Wall Bicep Curls
- **Cool-Down:** Wall Supported
Calf Raises, Wall-Assisted Seated
Piriformis Stretch, Wall
Supported Cat-Cow

Day 7: Rest Day

Week 3

Day 1: Flexibility and Core

- **Warm-Up:** Wall Hamstrings
Stretch, Wall Cat-Cow, Wall Arm
Circles
- **ABS and Core Exercise:** Wall
Plank, Modified Wall Plank, Wall
Knee Pulls
- **Cool-Down:** Wall Supported
Forward Fold, Wall-Assisted
Downward-Facing Dog, Wall Side
Bends

Day 2: Arms and Shoulders

- **Warm-Up:** Wall Heel Slides,
Wall Lateral Arm Raises, Wall
Chest Openers
- **Arms and Shoulder Exercise:**
Wall Arm Circles, Wall Diagonal
Arm Raises, Wall Bicep Curls
- **Cool-Down:** Wall Supported
Calf Raises, Wall-Assisted Seated
Piriformis Stretch, Wall
Supported Cat-Cow

Day 3: Lower Body

- **Warm-Up:** Wall Leg Lifts, Wall
Piriformis Stretch, Wall Neck
Rolls
- **Lower Body Exercise:** Wall
Squats, Modified Wall Squats,
Wall Calf Raises
- **Cool-Down:** Wall Single Leg
Raises, Wall Side Leg Lifts, Wall
Hip Abduction

Day 4: Flexibility and Balance

- **Warm-Up:** Wall Hamstrings

Stretch, Wall Side Bends, Wall Piriformis Stretch

- **Flexibility and Balance Exercise:** Wall Ankle Circles, Wall Single Leg Stands, Wall Heel-Toe Walk
- **Cool-Down:** Wall Cat-Cow, Deep Breaths

Day 5: Flexibility and Core

- **Warm-Up:** Wall Hamstrings Stretch, Wall Cat-Cow, Wall Arm Circles
- **ABS and Core Exercise:** Wall Plank, Modified Wall Plank, Wall Knee Pulls
- **Cool-Down:** Wall Supported Forward Fold, Wall-Assisted Downward-Facing Dog, Wall Side Bends

Day 6: Arms and Shoulders

- **Warm-Up:** Wall Heel Slides, Wall Lateral Arm Raises, Wall Chest Openers
- **Arms and Shoulder Exercise:** Wall Arm Circles, Wall Diagonal Arm Raises, Wall Bicep Curls
- **Cool-Down:** Wall Supported Calf Raises, Wall-Assisted Seated Piriformis Stretch, Wall Supported Cat-Cow

Day 7: Rest Day

Week 4

Day 1: Flexibility and Core

- **Warm-Up:** Wall Hamstrings Stretch, Wall Cat-Cow, Wall Arm Circles
- **ABS and Core Exercise:** Wall Plank, Modified Wall Plank, Wall Knee Pulls
- **Cool-Down:** Wall Supported Forward Fold, Wall-Assisted Downward-Facing Dog, Wall Side Bends

Day 2: Arms and Shoulders

- **Warm-Up:** Wall Heel Slides, Wall Lateral Arm Raises, Wall Chest Openers
- **Arms and Shoulder Exercise:** Wall Arm Circles, Wall Diagonal Arm Raises, Wall Bicep Curls
- **Cool-Down:** Wall Supported Calf Raises, Wall-Assisted Seated Piriformis Stretch, Wall Supported Cat-Cow

Day 3: Lower Body

- **Warm-Up:** Wall Leg Lifts, Wall Piriformis Stretch, Wall Neck Rolls
- **Lower Body Exercise:** Wall Squats, Modified Wall Squats, Wall Calf Raises
- **Cool-Down:** Wall Single Leg Raises, Wall Side Leg Lifts, Wall Hip Abduction

Weight Loss Weekly Workout Plan

Day 4: Flexibility and Balance

- **Warm-Up:** Wall Hamstrings Stretch, Wall Side Bends, Wall Piriformis Stretch
- **Flexibility and Balance Exercise:** Wall Ankle Circles, Wall Single Leg Stands, Wall Heel-Toe Walk
- **Cool-Down:** Wall Cat-Cow, Deep Breaths

Day 5: Flexibility and Core

- **Warm-Up:** Wall Hamstrings Stretch, Wall Cat-Cow, Wall Arm Circles
- **ABS and Core Exercise:** Wall Plank, Modified Wall Plank, Wall Knee Pulls
- **Cool-Down:** Wall Supported Forward Fold, Wall-Assisted Downward-Facing Dog, Wall Side Bends

Day 6: Arms and Shoulders

- **Warm-Up:** Wall Heel Slides, Wall Lateral Arm Raises, Wall Chest Openers
- **Arms and Shoulder Exercise:** Wall Arm Circles, Wall Diagonal Arm Raises, Wall Bicep Curls
- **Cool-Down:** Wall Supported Calf Raises, Wall-Assisted Seated Piriformis Stretch, Wall Supported Cat-Cow

Day 7: Rest Day

Day 1: Cardio and Core
30 minutes of brisk walking or jogging
ABS and Core Exercise: Bicycle Crunches, Plank, Russian Twists (3 sets of 12-15 reps)
Cool-Down: Stretching for 10 minutes

Day 2: Strength Training
Squats: 3 sets of 12 reps
Push-Ups: 3 sets of 10 reps
Lunges: 3 sets of 12 reps each leg
Bent-Over Rows: 3 sets of 12 reps
Cool-Down: Stretching for 10 minutes

Day 3: Cardio and Flexibility
30 minutes of cycling or swimming
Flexibility Exercise: Hamstring Stretch, Quadriceps Stretch, Shoulder Stretch (Hold each stretch for 30 seconds, repeat 2 times)
Cool-Down: Yoga for 10 minutes

Day 4: Active Rest
Light walking or cycling for 30 minutes
Gentle stretching for 10 minutes

Day 5: HIIT Workout
High-Intensity Interval Training (HIIT): 20 minutes (Alternate between 30 seconds of high-intensity exercise and 1 minute of rest)
ABS and Core Exercise: Plank Jacks, Mountain Climbers, Leg Raises (3 sets of 12-15 reps)

Cool-Down: Stretching for 10 minutes

Day 6: Strength Training

Deadlifts: 3 sets of 10 reps
Bench Press: 3 sets of 10 reps
Dumbbell Shoulder Press: 3 sets of 12 reps
Tricep Dips: 3 sets of 12 reps
Cool-Down: Stretching for 10 minutes

Day 7: Rest Day

Active recovery such as gentle walking or yoga for 30 minutes
Foam rolling for 10 minutes to release tension

Week 2

Day 1: Cardio and Core

40 minutes of brisk walking or jogging
ABS and Core Exercise: Russian Twists, Plank, Bicycle Crunches (3 sets of 15-20 reps)
Cool-Down: Stretching for 10 minutes

Day 2: Strength Training

Squats: 4 sets of 12 reps
Push-Ups: 4 sets of 10 reps
Lunges: 4 sets of 12 reps each leg
Bent-Over Rows: 4 sets of 12 reps
Cool-Down: Stretching for 10 minutes

Day 3: Cardio and Flexibility

40 minutes of cycling or swimming
Flexibility Exercise: Hamstring Stretch, Quadriceps Stretch, Shoulder Stretch (Hold each stretch for 30 seconds, repeat 3 times)
Cool-Down: Yoga for 15 minutes

Day 4: Active Rest

Light walking or cycling for 40 minutes
Gentle stretching for 15 minutes

Day 5: HIIT Workout

High-Intensity Interval Training (HIIT): 25 minutes (Alternate between 30 seconds of high-intensity exercise and 45 seconds of rest)
ABS and Core Exercise: Mountain Climbers, Plank Jacks, Leg Raises (3 sets of 15-20 reps)
Cool-Down: Stretching for 10 minutes

Day 6: Strength Training

Deadlifts: 4 sets of 10 reps
Bench Press: 4 sets of 10 reps
Dumbbell Shoulder Press: 4 sets of 12 reps
Tricep Dips: 4 sets of 12 reps
Cool-Down: Stretching for 10 minutes

Day 7: Rest Day

Active recovery such as gentle walking or yoga for 40 minutes
Foam rolling for 15 minutes to release tension

Week 3

Day 1: Cardio and Core

45 minutes of brisk walking or jogging
ABS and Core Exercise: Russian Twists, Plank, Bicycle Crunches (3 sets of 20-25 reps)
Cool-Down: Stretching for 10 minutes

Day 2: Strength Training

Squats: 4 sets of 12 reps
Push-Ups: 4 sets of 12 reps
Lunges: 4 sets of 12 reps each leg
Bent-Over Rows: 4 sets of 12 reps
Cool-Down: Stretching for 10 minutes

Day 3: Cardio and Flexibility

45 minutes of cycling or swimming
Flexibility Exercise: Hamstring Stretch, Quadriceps Stretch, Shoulder Stretch (Hold each stretch for 30 seconds, repeat 3 times)
Cool-Down: Yoga for 15 minutes

Day 4: Active Rest

Light walking or cycling for 45 minutes
Gentle stretching for 15 minutes

Day 5: HIIT Workout

High-Intensity Interval Training (HIIT): 30 minutes (Alternate between 30 seconds of high-intensity exercise and 30 seconds of rest)
ABS and Core Exercise: Mountain Climbers, Plank Jacks, Leg Raises (3 sets of 20-25 reps)
Cool-Down: Stretching for 10 minutes

Day 6: Strength Training

Deadlifts: 4 sets of 10 reps
Bench Press: 4 sets of 10 reps
Dumbbell Shoulder Press: 4 sets of 12 reps
Tricep Dips: 4 sets of 12 reps
Cool-Down: Stretching for 10 minutes

Day 7: Rest Day

Active recovery such as gentle walking or yoga for 45 minutes
Foam rolling for 15 minutes to release tension

Week 4

Day 1: Cardio and Core

50 minutes of brisk walking or jogging
ABS and Core Exercise: Russian Twists, Plank, Bicycle Crunches (3 sets of 20-25 reps)
Cool-Down: Stretching for 10 minutes

Day 2: Strength Training

Squats: 4 sets of 12 reps
Push-Ups: 4 sets of 12 reps
Lunges: 4 sets of 12 reps each leg
Bent-Over Rows: 4 sets of 12 reps
Cool-Down: Stretching for 10 minutes

Day 3: Cardio and Flexibility

50 minutes of cycling or swimming
Flexibility Exercise: Hamstring Stretch, Quadriceps Stretch, Shoulder Stretch (Hold each stretch for 30 seconds, repeat 3 times)
Cool-Down: Yoga for 15 minutes

Day 4: Active Rest

Light walking or cycling for 50 minutes
Gentle stretching for 15 minutes

Day 5: HIIT Workout

High-Intensity Interval Training (HIIT): 35 minutes (Alternate between 30 seconds of high-intensity exercise and 30 seconds of rest)
ABS and Core Exercise: Mountain Climbers, Plank Jacks, Leg Raises (3

| sets of 20-25 reps) |
| Cool-Down: Stretching for 10 minutes |
| |
| **Day 6: Strength Training** |
| |
| Deadlifts: 4 sets of 10 reps |
| Bench Press: 4 sets of 10 reps |
| Dumbbell Shoulder Press: 4 sets of 12 reps |
| Tricep Dips: 4 sets of 12 reps |
| Cool-Down: Stretching for 10 minutes |
| |
| **Day 7: Rest Day** |
| |
| Active recovery such as gentle walking or yoga for 50 minutes |
| Foam rolling for 15 minutes to release tension |

Core Strength & Flat Stomach Weekly Workout Plan

Week 1

Day 1: Core Activation

- **Warm-Up:** 10 minutes of brisk walking or jogging
- **Core Activation:** Plank Hold (3 sets, aim for 30 seconds each), Bicycle Crunches (3 sets of 15 reps), Russian Twists (3 sets of 15 reps)
- **Cool-Down:** Stretching focusing on the core muscles for 10 minutes

Day 2: Pilates for Core

- **Warm-Up:** 5 minutes of dynamic stretching
- **Pilates Core Exercises:** Hundred, Leg Lifts, Pilates Crunches (3 sets of 12 reps each)
- **Cool-Down:** 10 minutes of yoga focusing on the core muscles

Day 3: Cardio & Core

- **Cardio:** 20 minutes of interval training (alternate between 1 minute of high-intensity running or cycling and 1 minute of walking)
- **Core Workout:** Plank with Knee Tucks (3 sets of 12 reps), Mountain Climbers (3 sets of 15 reps each leg), Side Planks (3 sets of 30 seconds each side)
- **Cool-Down:** Stretching for 10 minutes

Day 4: Rest & Recovery

- Active recovery such as light walking or swimming for 30 minutes
- Foam rolling or gentle stretching for 15 minutes to aid recovery

Day 5: Total Core Blast

- **Warm-Up:** 5 minutes of dynamic stretching
- **Total Core Exercises:** V-Ups, Russian Twists with Medicine Ball (3 sets of 15 reps each side),

Plank with Hip Dips (3 sets of 12 reps)

- **Cool-Down:** 10 minutes of yoga focusing on core flexibility

Day 6: Pilates Core Strengthening

- **Warm-Up:** 10 minutes of brisk walking
- **Pilates Core Strengthening:** Roll-Ups, Double Leg Stretch, Teaser (3 sets of 10 reps each)
- **Cool-Down:** Stretching for 10 minutes

Day 7: Rest & Recovery

Complete rest day or light activity such as leisurely walking or gentle yoga for relaxation

Week 2

Day 1: Core Activation

- **Warm-Up:** 10 minutes of dynamic stretching
- **Core Activation:** Plank Hold (3 sets, aim for 45 seconds each), Bicycle Crunches (3 sets of 20 reps), Russian Twists with Medicine Ball (3 sets of 15 reps)
- **Cool-Down:** Stretching focusing on the core muscles for 10 minutes

Day 2: Pilates for Core

- **Warm-Up:** 5 minutes of brisk walking
- **Pilates Core Exercises:** Hundred, Leg Circles, Criss-Cross (3 sets of 15 reps each)
- **Cool-Down:** 10 minutes of yoga focusing on the core muscles

Day 3: Cardio & Core

- **Cardio:** 25 minutes of interval training (alternate between 1 minute of high-intensity running or cycling and 1 minute of walking)
- **Core Workout:** Plank with Knee Tucks (3 sets of 15 reps), Mountain Climbers (3 sets of 20 reps each leg), Side Planks with Rotation (3 sets of 12 reps each side)
- **Cool-Down:** Stretching for 10 minutes

Day 4: Rest & Recovery

Active recovery such as light walking or swimming for 30 minutes
Foam rolling or gentle stretching for 15 minutes to aid recovery

Day 5: Total Core Blast

- **Warm-Up:** 5 minutes of dynamic stretching
- **Total Core Exercises:** Hanging Leg Raises, Russian Twists with Medicine Ball (3 sets of 20 reps each side), Plank with Hip Dips (3 sets of 15 reps)

- **Cool-Down:** 10 minutes of yoga focusing on core flexibility

Day 6: Pilates Core Strengthening

- **Warm-Up:** 10 minutes of brisk walking
- **Pilates Core Strengthening:** Roll-Ups, Scissors, Corkscrew (3 sets of 12 reps each)
- **Cool-Down:** Stretching for 10 minutes

Day 7: Rest & Recovery

Complete rest day or light activity such as leisurely walking or gentle yoga for relaxation

Week 3

Day 1: Core Activation

- **Warm-Up:** 10 minutes of dynamic stretching
- **Core Activation:** Plank Hold (3 sets, aim for 1 minute each), Bicycle Crunches (3 sets of 25 reps), Russian Twists with Medicine Ball (3 sets of 20 reps)
- **Cool-Down:** Stretching focusing on the core muscles for 10 minutes

Day 2: Pilates for Core

- **Warm-Up:** 5 minutes of brisk walking
- **Pilates Core Exercises:** Hundred, Roll Like a Ball, Saw (3 sets of 15 reps each)
- **Cool-Down:** 10 minutes of yoga focusing on the core muscles

Day 3: Cardio & Core

- **Cardio:** 30 minutes of interval training (alternate between 1 minute of high-intensity running or cycling and 1 minute of walking)
- **Core Workout:** Plank with Knee Tucks (3 sets of 20 reps), Mountain Climbers (3 sets of 25 reps each leg), Side Planks with Rotation (3 sets of 15 reps each side)
- **Cool-Down:** Stretching for 10 minutes

Day 4: Rest & Recovery

Active recovery such as light walking or swimming for 30 minutes
Foam rolling or gentle stretching for 15 minutes to aid recovery

Day 5: Total Core Blast

- **Warm-Up:** 5 minutes of dynamic stretching
- **Total Core Exercises:** Hanging Leg Raises, Russian Twists with Medicine Ball (3 sets of 25 reps each side), Plank with Hip Dips (3 sets of 20 reps)
- **Cool-Down:** 10 minutes of yoga focusing on core flexibility

Day 6: Pilates Core Strengthening

- **Warm-Up:** 10 minutes of brisk walking
- **Pilates Core Strengthening:** Teaser, Side Leg Lift Series, Swimming (3 sets of 15 reps each)
- **Cool-Down:** Stretching for 10 minutes

Day 7: Rest & Recovery

Complete rest day or light activity such as leisurely walking or gentle yoga for relaxation

Week 4:

Day 1: Core Activation

- **Warm-Up:** 10 minutes of dynamic stretching
- **Core Activation:** Plank Hold (3 sets, aim for 1 minute each), Bicycle Crunches (3 sets of 30 reps), Russian Twists with Medicine Ball (3 sets of 25 reps)
- **Cool-Down:** Stretching focusing on the core muscles for 10 minutes

Day 2: Pilates for Core

- **Warm-Up:** 5 minutes of brisk walking
- **Pilates Core Exercises:** Hundred, Roll-Up to Teaser, Side Bend (3 sets of 20 reps each)

- **Cool-Down:** 10 minutes of yoga focusing on the core muscles

Day 3: Cardio & Core

- **Cardio:** 35 minutes of interval training (alternate between 1 minute of high-intensity running or cycling and 1 minute of walking)
- **Core Workout:** Plank with Knee Tucks (3 sets of 25 reps), Mountain Climbers (3 sets of 30 reps each leg), Side Planks with Rotation (3 sets of 20 reps each side)
- **Cool-Down:** Stretching for 10 minutes

Day 4: Rest & Recovery

Active recovery such as light walking or swimming for 30 minutes
Foam rolling or gentle stretching for 15 minutes to aid recovery

Day 5: Total Core Blast

- **Warm-Up:** 5 minutes of dynamic stretching
- **Total Core Exercises:** Hanging Leg Raises, Russian Twists with Medicine Ball (3 sets of 30 reps each side), Plank with Hip Dips (3 sets of 25 reps)
- **Cool-Down:** 10 minutes of yoga focusing on core flexibility

Day 6: Pilates Core Strengthening

- **Warm-Up:** 10 minutes of brisk walking
- **Pilates Core Strengthening:** Corkscrew, Side Plank with Leg Lift, Scissors (3 sets of 20 reps each)
- **Cool-Down:** Stretching for 10 minutes

Day 7: Rest & Recovery

Complete rest day or light activity such as leisurely walking or gentle yoga for relaxation

28 days Challenges

Day 1: Core and Balance Focus

Wall Plank - Hold for 1 minute, repeat 3 times
Modified Wall Plank - Hold for 45 seconds, repeat 3 times
Wall Knee Pulls - 15 reps each leg, 3 sets
Wall Side Leg Lifts - 15 reps each leg, 3 sets
Wall Single Leg Stands - Hold for 30 seconds each leg, repeat 3 times

Day 2: Upper Body Strength

Wall Arm Circles - 20 reps forward, 20 reps backward, 3 sets
Wall Bicep Curls - 15 reps, 3 sets
Wall Lateral Arm Raises - 15 reps each arm, 3 sets
Wall Tricep Extensions - 15 reps, 3 sets
Wall Shoulder Rolls - 20 reps, 3 sets

Day 3: Lower Body Power

Wall Squats with Calf Raise - 15 reps, 3 sets
Wall Lunges - 10 reps each leg, 3 sets
Wall Leg Lifts - 15 reps each leg, 3 sets
Wall Heel Slides - 15 reps each leg, 3 sets
Wall Hip Abduction - 15 reps each leg, 3 sets

Day 4: Flexibility and Mobility

Wall Hamstring Stretch - Hold for 1 minute, repeat 3 times
Wall Piriformis Stretch - Hold for 30 seconds each side, repeat 3 times
Wall Ankle Circles - 20 circles each direction, 3 sets
Wall Neck Rolls - 10 reps each direction, 3 sets
Wall Cat-Cow with Modifications - 15 reps, 3 sets

Day 5: Cardio and Core Blast

Wall Mountain Climbers - 20 reps each leg, 3 sets
Wall Plank Jacks - 15 reps, 3 sets
Wall Russian Twists - 20 reps each side, 3 sets
Wall Knee Tucks - 15 reps, 3 sets
Wall Burpees - 10 reps, 3 sets

Day 6: Balance and Stability

| Wall Single Leg Stands with Eyes Closed - Hold for 30 seconds each leg, repeat 3 sets |
| Wall Heel-Toe Walk - 10 steps forward, 10 steps backward, 3 sets |
| Wall Side Bends - 15 reps each side, 3 sets |
| Wall Single Leg Raises - 15 reps each leg, 3 sets |
| Wall Supported March - 20 reps each leg, 3 sets |

Day 7: Active Recovery

Enjoy a day of active recovery such as swimming, walking, or gentle yoga to rejuvenate your body and mind.

Day 8: Core and Balance Focus

| Wall Plank with Leg Lifts - Hold for 1 minute, lift one leg at a time for 10 reps each, repeat 3 sets |
| Wall Side Plank with Hip Dips - Hold side plank for 45 seconds each side, dip hip towards floor and raise back up, 10 reps each side, repeat 3 sets |
| Wall Russian Twists with Medicine Ball - 20 reps each side, 3 sets |
| Wall Crunches with Twist - 15 reps each side, 3 sets |
| Wall Knee Tucks with Rotation - 15 reps each side, 3 sets |

Day 9: Upper Body Endurance

| Wall Push-Ups with Rotation - 15 reps, alternating sides, 3 sets |
| Wall Tricep Dips - 15 reps, 3 sets |
| Wall Shoulder Press - 15 reps, 3 sets |

| Wall Arm Circles with Resistance Band - 20 reps forward, 20 reps backward, 3 sets |
| Wall Bicep Curls with Resistance Band - 15 reps, 3 sets |

Day 10: Lower Body Burn

| Wall Squats with Pulse - 15 reps, pulse at the bottom for 10 seconds, 3 sets |
| Wall Bulgarian Split Squats - 10 reps each leg, 3 sets |
| Wall Calf Raises with Resistance Band - 20 reps, 3 sets |
| Wall Side Leg Lifts with Resistance Band - 15 reps each leg, 3 sets |
| Wall Hip Abduction with Resistance Band - 15 reps each leg, 3 sets |

Day 11: Flexibility and Mobility

| Wall Hamstring Stretch with Resistance Band - Hold for 1 minute, repeat 3 times |
| Wall Quadriceps Stretch - Hold for 45 seconds each leg, repeat 3 times |
| Wall Figure Four Stretch - Hold for 45 seconds each leg, repeat 3 times |
| Wall Chest Opener Stretch - Hold for 45 seconds, repeat 3 times |
| Wall Shoulder Stretch - Hold for 45 seconds each arm, repeat 3 times |

Day 12: Cardio and Core Fusion

| Wall Mountain Climbers - 20 reps each leg, 3 sets |
| Wall Plank Jacks - 15 reps, 3 sets |
| Wall Sprinters - 15 reps each leg, 3 sets |

Wall Burpees - 10 reps, 3 sets	reps each side, 4 sets
Wall Bicycle Crunches - 20 reps each side, 3 sets	**Wall Knee Tucks with Rotation** - 20 reps each side, 4 sets

Day 13: Balance and Stability

Wall Single Leg Stands with Resistance Band - Hold for 45 seconds each leg, repeat 3 sets

Wall Heel-Toe Walk with Resistance Band - 15 steps forward, 15 steps backward, 3 sets

Wall Side Bends with Resistance Band - 15 reps each side, 3 sets

Wall Single Leg Raises with Resistance Band - 15 reps each leg, 3 sets

Wall Supported March with Resistance Band - 20 reps each leg, 3 sets

Day 14: Active Recovery

Engage in a day of light activity such as swimming, walking, or gentle stretching to aid in recovery and prepare for the next week of challenges.

Day 15: Core and Balance Focus

Wall Plank with Leg Lifts - Hold for 1 minute, lift one leg at a time for 12 reps each, repeat 4 sets

Wall Side Plank with Hip Dips - Hold side plank for 45 seconds each side, dip hip towards floor and raise back up, 12 reps each side, repeat 4 sets

Wall Russian Twists with Medicine Ball - 25 reps each side, 4 sets

Wall Crunches with Twist - 20

Day 16: Upper Body Endurance

Wall Push-Ups with Rotation - 18 reps, alternating sides, 4 sets

Wall Tricep Dips - 18 reps, 4 sets

Wall Shoulder Press - 18 reps, 4 sets

Wall Arm Circles with Resistance Band - 25 reps forward, 25 reps backward, 4 sets

Wall Bicep Curls with Resistance Band - 18 reps, 4 sets

Day 17: Lower Body Burn

Wall Squats with Pulse - 18 reps, pulse at the bottom for 15 seconds, 4 sets

Wall Bulgarian Split Squats - 12 reps each leg, 4 sets

Wall Calf Raises with Resistance Band - 25 reps, 4 sets

Wall Side Leg Lifts with Resistance Band - 18 reps each leg, 4 sets

Wall Hip Abduction with Resistance Band - 18 reps each leg, 4 sets

Day 18: Flexibility and Mobility

Wall Hamstring Stretch with Resistance Band - Hold for 1 minute, repeat 4 times

Wall Quadriceps Stretch - Hold for 1 minute each leg, repeat 4 times

Wall Figure Four Stretch - Hold for 1 minute each leg, repeat 4 times

Wall Chest Opener Stretch - Hold

for 1 minute, repeat 4 times

Wall Shoulder Stretch - Hold for 1 minute each arm, repeat 4 times

Day 19: Cardio and Core Fusion

Wall Mountain Climbers - 25 reps each leg, 4 sets

Wall Plank Jacks - 20 reps, 4 sets

Wall Sprinters - 20 reps each leg, 4 sets

Wall Burpees - 12 reps, 4 sets

Wall Bicycle Crunches - 25 reps each side, 4 sets

Day 20: Balance and Stability

Wall Single Leg Stands with Resistance Band - Hold for 1 minute each leg, repeat 4 sets

Wall Heel-Toe Walk with Resistance Band - 20 steps forward, 20 steps backward, 4 sets

Wall Side Bends with Resistance Band - 20 reps each side, 4 sets

Wall Single Leg Raises with Resistance Band - 20 reps each leg, 4 sets

Wall Supported March with Resistance Band - 25 reps each leg, 4 sets

Day 21: Active Recovery

Engage in a day of light activity such as swimming, walking, or gentle stretching to aid in recovery and prepare for the next week of challenges.

Day 22: Core and Balance Focus

Wall Plank with Leg Lifts - Hold for 1 minute, lift one leg at a time for 15 reps each, repeat 4 sets

Wall Side Plank with Hip Dips - Hold side plank for 1 minute each side, dip hip towards floor and raise back up, 15 reps each side, repeat 4 sets

Wall Russian Twists with Medicine Ball - 30 reps each side, 4 sets

Wall Crunches with Twist - 25 reps each side, 4 sets

Wall Knee Tucks with Rotation - 25 reps each side, 4 sets

Day 23: Upper Body Endurance

Wall Push-Ups with Rotation - 20 reps, alternating sides, 4 sets

Wall Tricep Dips - 20 reps, 4 sets

Wall Shoulder Press - 20 reps, 4 sets

Wall Arm Circles with Resistance Band - 30 reps forward, 30 reps backward, 4 sets

Wall Bicep Curls with Resistance Band - 20 reps, 4 sets

Day 24: Lower Body Burn

Wall Squats with Pulse - 20 reps, pulse at the bottom for 15 seconds, 4 sets

Wall Bulgarian Split Squats - 15 reps each leg, 4 sets

Wall Calf Raises with Resistance Band - 30 reps, 4 sets

Wall Side Leg Lifts with Resistance Band - 20 reps each leg, 4 sets

Wall Hip Abduction with Resistance Band - 20 reps each leg, 4 sets

Day 25: Flexibility and Mobility

Wall Hamstring Stretch with Resistance Band - Hold for 1.5 minutes, repeat 4 times

Wall Quadriceps Stretch - Hold for 1.5 minutes each leg, repeat 4 times

Wall Figure Four Stretch - Hold for 1.5 minutes each leg, repeat 4 times

Wall Chest Opener Stretch - Hold for 1.5 minutes, repeat 4 times

Wall Shoulder Stretch - Hold for 1.5 minutes each arm, repeat 4 times

Day 26: Cardio and Core Fusion

Wall Mountain Climbers - 30 reps each leg, 4 sets

Wall Plank Jacks - 25 reps, 4 sets

Wall Sprinters - 25 reps each leg, 4 sets

Wall Burpees - 15 reps, 4 sets

Wall Bicycle Crunches - 30 reps each side, 4 sets

Day 27: Balance and Stability

Wall Single Leg Stands with Resistance Band - Hold for 1.5 minutes each leg, repeat 4 sets

Wall Heel-Toe Walk with Resistance Band - 25 steps forward, 25 steps backward, 4 sets

Wall Side Bends with Resistance Band - 25 reps each side, 4 sets

Wall Single Leg Raises with Resistance Band - 25 reps each leg, 4 sets

Wall Supported March with Resistance Band - 30 reps each leg, 4 sets

Day 28: Active Recovery

Engage in a day of light activity such as swimming, walking, or gentle stretching to aid in recovery and prepare for the next week of challenges.

7

NUTRITION AID WELL BEING

Nutritional Tips for Optimal Performance In Wall Pilate

Pilates exercises offer a wide range of benefits, including enhanced flexibility, toned muscles throughout the body, improved balance, and increased mobility. The impact of Pilates can be further optimized by fueling your body with appropriate nutrients.

Timing your pre-workout meals is crucial to ensure optimal performance during your Pilates class. Consuming a heavy meal shortly before class can lead to discomfort and hinder your performance. While the ideal timing may vary for each individual, it's generally recommended to avoid eating within an hour of your session, with a preferable gap of two hours between eating and exercising.

Experiment with different timings and food combinations to find what works best for your body.

Selecting the right foods before a Pilates class is essential to maintain energy levels without feeling too full or sluggish. Here are some guidelines to consider:

- Avoid foods that may cause bloating or gas, such as cabbage, onions, lentils, beans, cauliflower, broccoli, and garlic.
- Steer clear of heavy or slow-to-digest meals.
- Minimize consumption of sugary or high-carb foods.
- Opt for light meals or snacks containing healthy fats, lean protein, and complex carbohydrates to sustain energy levels and support performance.

For morning classes, choose lighter options like yogurt with nuts and berries or a banana with nut butter. For afternoon sessions, consider energy-dense meals such as an omelette with avocado or a salad with lean protein.

Here are some examples of pre-workout snacks and meals suitable for Pilates:

- Scrambled eggs with avocado and berries
- Unsweetened yogurt with berries and nuts
- Apple slices with nut butter and cheese
- Leafy green salad with nuts and boiled egg
- Lettuce wrap with sliced turkey
- Banana with almond butter
- Celery sticks with hummus
- Green smoothie with leafy greens, fruit, and yogurt
- High-quality protein bar or shake
- Oatmeal with berries
- Nut butter on whole grain toast with baby carrots or berries

After your Pilates class, aim to consume a small meal or snack within 30 to 60 minutes to replenish glycogen stores and provide your muscles with the necessary nutrients for recovery and repair.

After completing a Pilates class, it's essential to refuel your body with a balanced combination of lean protein, healthy fats, and complex carbohydrates.

Here are some nutritious and convenient post-Pilates meal suggestions:

- Blend a protein shake using high-quality protein powder and wholesome ingredients.
- Enjoy a serving of plain Greek yogurt topped with fresh fruit and nuts.
- Indulge in a bowl of oatmeal topped with berries, accompanied by a boiled egg.
- Prepare a veggie-packed omelette filled with spinach, asparagus, onions, mushrooms, bell peppers, and black olives, finished with diced avocado.
- Pair sweet potatoes with a serving of fish or grilled chicken for a satisfying meal.
- Serve grilled chicken alongside brown rice and non-starchy vegetables.
- Create a hearty salad featuring diced boiled egg, pistachios, bell pepper, sunflower seeds, and assorted vegetables of your choice.

- Savor a nourishing bean soup loaded with vegetables, accompanied by a slice of sprouted whole-grain bread.
- Whip up a nutrient-rich smoothie with yogurt, berries, a scoop of nut butter, and a handful of spinach.

Maintaining a balanced diet between Pilates sessions is crucial for achieving long, lean muscles and sustaining consistent energy levels.

Include the following nutrient-dense foods in your diet:

- Nuts, seeds, and nut butter
- Healthy fats from wild-caught fish like salmon, sardines, tuna, and anchovies
- Unsweetened yogurt
- Fresh fruits and vegetables
- Leafy greens
- Whole grains such as oats, millet, brown rice, barley, and quinoa
- Lean protein sources like chicken, turkey, fish, full-fat dairy, and eggs

Moderation is key, so allow yourself occasional indulgences to maintain balance and promote long-term success.

Hydration is crucial to support your body's function and performance during Pilates workouts. Ensure you drink enough fluids before, during, and after exercise to prevent fatigue, enhance concentration, and maintain optimal body function.

Drink at least one 8-ounce glass of water 30 minutes before your Pilates class and keep a water bottle nearby to sip during the session. Afterward, replenish lost fluids by consuming at least two cups of water within 30 minutes to an hour post-workout. Fruits and vegetables with high water content can also contribute to your hydration needs.

While Pilates can be challenging, it typically doesn't require extensive carbohydrate consumption like endurance activities or intense workouts. While eating some healthy carbs before class can provide sustained energy, excessive carb loading is unnecessary.

Sports drinks are generally not needed for Pilates sessions, as they're not as intense or prolonged as other forms of exercise. If you choose to consume a sports drink, opt for options with minimal added sugars to avoid unnecessary calorie intake.

Micronutrient and Their Sources

Micronutrients play a vital role in supporting overall health and well-being, especially for individuals engaging in physical activities like Wall Pilates. Here's a breakdown of essential micronutrients and their food sources suitable for seniors and beginners:

Vitamin A:

Sources: Sweet potatoes, carrots, spinach, kale, squash, apricots, and fortified dairy products.
Benefits: Supports vision, immune function, and skin health.

Vitamin C:

Sources: Citrus fruits (oranges, lemons), strawberries, bell peppers, broccoli, kiwi, and tomatoes.
Benefits: Boosts immune function, aids in collagen production, and acts as an antioxidant.

Vitamin D:

Sources: Fatty fish (salmon, mackerel), fortified dairy products, egg yolks, and exposure to sunlight.
Benefits: Supports bone health, immune function, and mood regulation.

Vitamin E:

Sources: Nuts (almonds, hazelnuts), seeds (sunflower seeds), spinach, broccoli, and vegetable oils.
Benefits: Acts as an antioxidant, protects cells from damage, and supports immune function.

Vitamin K:

Sources: Leafy greens (spinach, kale, Swiss chard), broccoli, Brussels sprouts, and green peas.

Benefits: Essential for blood clotting, bone health, and cardiovascular health.
B Vitamins (B1, B2, B3, B5, B6, B7, B9, B12):

Sources: Whole grains, lean meats, poultry, fish, eggs, dairy products, legumes, nuts, seeds, and leafy greens.
Benefits: Essential for energy metabolism, nerve function, red blood cell production, and brain health.

Calcium:

Sources: Dairy products (milk, yogurt, cheese), fortified plant-based milk, tofu, almonds, leafy greens (kale, collard greens), and canned fish with bones (sardines, salmon).
Benefits: Crucial for bone health, muscle function, nerve transmission, and blood clotting.

Magnesium:

Sources: Nuts (almonds, cashews), seeds (pumpkin seeds, sunflower seeds), whole grains, leafy greens, legumes, and dark chocolate.
Benefits: Supports muscle and nerve function, regulates blood sugar levels, and contributes to bone health.

Iron:

Sources: Lean meats, poultry, fish, legumes (beans, lentils), tofu, spinach, fortified cereals, and pumpkin seeds.

Benefits: Necessary for oxygen transport, energy metabolism, and immune function.

Zinc:

Sources: Shellfish (oysters, crab), red meat, poultry, beans, nuts, seeds, whole grains, and dairy products.
Benefits: Supports immune function, wound healing, and protein synthesis.
Incorporating a balanced diet rich in these micronutrients can enhance energy levels, support muscle function, aid in recovery, and promote overall health for individuals participating in Wall Pilates, regardless of their age or fitness level.

CONCLUSION

As we reach the final chapter of "Wall Pilates for Seniors and Beginners," it's a moment to reflect on the incredible journey we've embarked upon together. Throughout these pages, we've explored the transformative power of Wall Pilates—a gentle yet profound practice that has the potential to reshape our bodies, minds, and lives.

From the foundational stretches to the challenging exercises, we've delved into the core principles of Wall Pilates, discovering how it can enhance flexibility, build strength, and improve overall well-being. With each movement, each breath, we've cultivated a deeper connection to ourselves, unlocking our innate potential for growth and healing.

But beyond the physical benefits, Wall Pilates has offered us something even more valuable—a sense of community, support, and shared purpose. In the camaraderie of our fellow practitioners, we've found encouragement, inspiration, and a shared commitment to health and vitality.

As we prepare to close this chapter, let us carry with us the lessons learned and the memories cherished. Let us continue to embrace the principles of Wall Pilates in our daily lives, using its teachings to navigate the challenges and triumphs that lie ahead.

With gratitude for the journey, we've shared and anticipation for the adventures yet to come, let us bid farewell to this book, knowing that its wisdom will remain with us always.

May we move forward with strength, resilience, and a renewed sense of purpose, knowing that the practice of Wall Pilates has equipped us with the tools we need to thrive in body, mind, and spirit.

Thank you for joining me on this transformative journey. Until we meet again on the mat, may your practice be filled with joy, vitality, and boundless possibility.

www.ingramcontent.com/pod-product-compliance
Lightning Source LLC
Chambersburg PA
CBHW081221260726
48653CB00010BB/3738

* 9 7 9 8 3 2 5 0 3 8 4 4 0 *